EDGAR CAYCE AND THE

Yoga Sutras

EDGAR CAYCE AND THE

Yoga Sutras

❦

Uniting Body, Mind, and Spirit

Istvan Fazekas

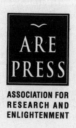

~
ARE
PRESS

**ASSOCIATION FOR
RESEARCH AND
ENLIGHTENMENT**

A.R.E. Press • Virginia Beach • Virginia

A.R.E. Press
215 67th Street
Virginia Beach, VA 23451–2061

Fazekas, Istvan, 1964–.
    Edgar Cayce and the Yoga sutras : uniting body, mind, and spirit / by Istvan Fazekas.
        p.   cm.
    Includes bibliographical references. (p.   ).
    ISBN 978-0-87604-530-5 (trade paper)
    1. Cayce, Edgar, 1877–1945. Edgar Cayce readings. 2. Patañjali. Yogasutra.
3. Yoga, Raja. I. Title.
    BF1045.Y63F39 2008
    133.8092—dc22

                                                2008044718

The author gratefully acknowledges the following publishers for permission to re-print sayings throughout the book:

Crystal Clarity Publishers, www.crystalclarity.com. *Conversations with Yogananda* by Swami Kriyananda.

Self-Realization Fellowship, Los Angeles, CA. The sayings of Paramahansa Yogananda in *The Divine Romance, God Talks with Arjuna,* and *Man's Eternal Quest.*

Ramakrishna–Vivekananda Center of New York. *The Gospel of Sri Ramakrishna,* as translated into English by Swami Nikhilananda, copyright 1942, and *Vivekananda: The Yogas and Other Works* by Swami Nikhilananda, Trustee of the Estate of Swami Vivekananda, copyright 1953.

Cover design by Richard Boyle

To the greatest of all mahayogis:
Rabbi Yeshu'a ben Ab Elyon, Ha Notzri

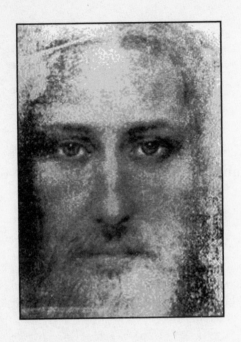

Mahayogi Yeshua

[T]o the uplift of India, that in which it has been and is so oft misunderstood . . . to the truths that India holds and has held that the world so much needs, in [the world's] mad rush for the expression of the desires of the flesh.

Edgar Cayce Reading 866-1

CONTENTS

Acknowledgments

It is a pleasure to record my gratitude to the many people who have made the journey to this endeavor possible, and for reasons too numerous to mention in detail. I would like to recognize first and foremost, my dear friend Ed Rocks, who left the body too soon for me to express my gratitude to him for all his friendship and inspiration. He saw my path years before I did. Thanks for everything, Rockdananda.

To Grethe Tedrick, who was the stalwart Northern California A.R.E. Region Coordinator when I first started doing various presentations and projects for the Region years ago, now retired, and Julie Hilt, the current sparkling light at the helm. Their encouragement continues to be greatly valued.

To Rev. Iclea Halton, a Mãe de Santo, shamana and friend. Obrigado minha amiga.

I must recognize the teacher who initially opened my mind at age twenty-one to spiritual truths, Jiddu Krishnamurti. At the time, his words were like none I had encountered before. And to the holy lights, the yogic masters, of whom I still gain inspiration and guidance and bow in reverence to their awesome accomplishments: Paramahansa Ramakrishna, Swami Vivekananda, Paramahansa Yogananda, Baba Hari Dass, Ramana Maharshi, Neem Karoli Baba, Jelaluddin Rumi, Hazrat Inayat Khan, Peace Pilgrim, and Jesus the Christ.

I must also thank Ram Dass (Dr. Richard Alpert), who showed me the value of taking risks. Even though fate substituted his prized sports car with a wheelchair, his bawdy humor and astute observations continue to be valuable fingers pointing at the moon.

Thanks to Nancy Eubel, Stephanie Hellberg, Suzun Almquist, Rick Gwyn, Ilona Marshall, Doug and Nancy Hilton, and all the Search for God Study Group members throughout the years.

To my mother, Joyce, for all her love and laughs; my sister, Sári, for her untiring encouragement; J. L. Goldman and Joe Quinn, both positive influences at crucial times; and dear Uncle Hefti (Imre Fazekas), for always rewarding knowledge and humor, while shunning intimidation.

A special thank you to Doris Van Auken at A.R.E. Press, who, like the

Buddhist counterpart to Saint Michael, Mahaboddhisatva Manjusri, wielded her editorial sword of wisdom with both compassion and insight to make this book presentable and coherent. Any shortcomings in those areas are solely the burden of the author, not the editor.

And last, to all the wonderful friends and relationships that have each taught me something about myself—I treasure every one. The learning continues ad infinitum . . . until the yoga is perfected.

Everywhere you go, there you are—
so, where are you going?
—Istvan Fazekas

◆

Foreword

This is a book about love—in the purest sense of the word—the unconditional love the Creator has for its creation, and the principles for
opening ourselves to *experience* that love in a more expansive and fulfilling way. There is no better time for this spiritual awakening than now,
according to Istvan Fazekas, not in the future, not in 2012. Moreover, as
Eckhart Tolle reminds us in his bestselling book *A New Earth*, which has
swept the country, when humanity in the past looked to some future
event for salvation or awakening, it *missed the moment*—and the present
moment, as we have come to realize, is all we have.

The spiritual awakening and enlightenment we seek is not an intellectual pursuit but one of the soul's yearning for communion through
the heart and spirit—a hunger for a deeper sense of the Divine's presence in our lives. So it is that within these pages, Istvan gently moves
the reader from the conceptual and intellectual into the sacred mysticism of practical spiritual living, for only in the application of the
wisdom of the sages is spirituality made practical in the day-to-day

living of these changing times.

One of the first principles taught in the ancient mystery schools was *Know thyself.* Plato gave discourses on this principle. The twentieth-century mystic Edgar Cayce presented it as the second lesson in the Search For God Study Group readings. And Fazekas presents it as a fundamental step in self-transformation.

Through eons of time, spiritual teachers and masters have returned to earth to remind us of the all-important truth that we are the children of a Creator of Infinite Love. We uplift and actually transform the world when we move from the promptings of the heart to be channels for manifesting the unconditional love of God to others. Not through some great act, but just through being kind, compassionate, forgiving, and patient, lending encouragement to the discouraged . . . being positive in our thinking and our actions. And, most importantly, in recognizing the profound truth that we are not separate from one another or the Source we came from—hence we cannot do ill to another without it doing ill to ourselves and to our Maker.

Istvan has been a spiritual mentor to me. He has taught me a great deal about how to befriend, or embrace, those things that are uncomfortable or painful. Most of us can identify with a period in life when we ran away from our fear and pain. In my experience, those things I ran from were always waiting for me at the front door, no matter how fast or hard I ran. In this book, Istvan presents these challenges as soul-growth opportunities and gives illuminating examples of how we can fearlessly move forward, face our uncertainties and fears head-on, and embrace all of life's experiences—knowing always that there is a light at the end of the tunnel. In fact, through the passage of experience and being in the now, we can become "as lights to the waiting world," according to Cayce, by passing through our challenges and helping others. Istvan writes of this with clarity and with great compassion—like all of us, he has passed through many experiences, both light and dark. And, in truth, Istvan writes as he lives—from the heart. He is both delightfully human and artfully spiritual. He remains a source of great inspiration to me as a friend.

The book you hold in your hands is a testament of Istvan's simple desire to share what he has learned, to try to light the way for others by sharing the spiritual truths that have helped him in his trek through this world. Through that heartfelt desire and willingness to try to be of help, he follows in the footsteps of the masters.

Robert J. Grant
November 2008
Virginia Beach, Virginia

Life itself is the result of the Creator's love for humanity.
–Istvan Fazekas

Robert J. Grant is the author of the following books:
Edgar Cayce on Angels, Archangels, and the Unseen Forces
The Magdalene Diaries
The Place We Call Home: Exploring the Soul's Existence After Death
Universe of Worlds: Exploring the Frontiers of the Afterlife

Introduction

Years ago I realized the connection between the information presented in books I and II of *A Search for God* and the basic principles of Raja Yoga, the ancient science of God realization. Although not identical, there are many significant similarities, far too many for me to ignore. It is clear that the Cayce readings' source was pulling from a metaphysical reserve of established ideas common to many religions. Most of these were developed and systematized in a geographic triangle that stretched from India in the east to Egypt in the west to the regions of Kazakhstan in the north, past the Caspian Sea. In this area the roots of Judaism, Christianity, Islam, Buddhism, and Hinduism were all developed. The readings' source tapped into akashic ideas that touch upon many of these religions' ideological foundations.

It is also significant to know, as given through the readings' source, that the historical Jesus (Yeshua in Hebrew) was sent to India by his teacher Judy, the Essene priestess. The readings state that Judy was influenced by Asian philosophy, and this *had* to influence the young Yeshua, even before his travels to India, Persia, and Egypt. This knowledge is not part of standard Christian theological ideology, nor is reincarnation or other fascinating fragments of the historical Palestinian drama that we get from the readings. This is what may place this information in the "lunatic fringe" category in some people's estimation. But it is my firm belief that original Christianity, the kind that would have been imparted and endorsed by the historical Yeshua, before there was even such a sect as "Christianity," is much closer to Raja Yoga than to many popular ideologies that rely on mere rhetoric or blind obedience. Yeshua's teacher studied Asian beliefs, and he himself would do so as a young man. He certainly proved himself to be a yogi of the highest caliber—a mahayogi.

It is tragic that the mystical roots of Christianity have been systematically diluted, even erased, by sociopolitical factions over the last two thousand years. The contemporary American Christian creed and practice would not be recognizable or even remotely related to the practices of the early Palestinian Jews and Essenes. In some modern congregations, there is even a fallacious belief that yoga, in any form, is somehow a threat to Christian values. Anyone who takes the time to investigate the beautiful and sublime teachings of spiritual yoga will obviously see through the absurdity of this.

What is needed in this day and age is to restore an understanding of common spiritual unity and allow one another to worship as each sees appropriate, as long as individual methods do not violate the tenets found in the *yamas* and *niyamas*, the transreligious moral foundations for the world.

Christians, if they are truly such, should be the most faithful adherents to the teachings of the Christ—to forgive "seven times seventy"; to "love thy neighbor as thyself"; to find the "kingdom of God within"; to put away the sword because "those who live by the sword, die by the sword"; to serve all because "he who is chief among you shall be the servant of *all.*" If nothing else, each should stay faithful to Jesus' chief commandment to "Love one another as I have loved you." These tenets also align with many of the masters of India, Tibet, China, and Japan. From a spiritual perspective, they are all in perfect accord, even with their unique cultural distinctions.

If Jesus traveled through India, as the Cayce source states repeatedly and as numerous teachers in India have affirmed, then he certainly would have known of spiritual yoga. Jesus even uses the word *yoke*, the English translation of the Sanskrit *yoga*, in the following passage from Matthew's Gospel:

Take my yoke upon you, and learn of Me; for I am gentle (meek) and humble (lowly) in heart, and you will find rest . . . for your souls. For My yoke is wholesome (useful, good)—not harsh . . . or sharp, but comfortable, gracious, and pleasant; and My burden is light and easy to be borne.

Matthew 11:29-30 (The Amplified Bible)

In many ways, the readings' source outlined a type of Christian yoga, a metaphysical Christianity that transcends institutional limitations and leads the sincere seeker straight into the presence of the Divine by pragmatic means. This is also the offering of this book.

Eighteen hundred years ago a collection of pithy teachings, or *sutras*, was codified by a sage named Patañjali. The *Yoga Sutras* of Patañjali are regarded as one of the most important collections of concise wisdom on spiritual yoga and have been employed by sages for centuries as a step-by-step manual for consciousness transformation. This collection of sutras is not a substitute for studying with a God-realized sage but instead is used as an accompaniment. Interestingly enough, the same can be said of the *A Search for God* books, although the latter have a much shorter track record.

Anyone who over time has committed to studying the Search for God teachings in a study group format, putting into practice the lessons' recommendations and sifting through the sometimes difficult-to-decipher passages, can vouch for the true transformational power of the material. It is challenging at times, but it is supposed to be. It is Christ Consciousness yoga and likely the most important contribution the Cayce legacy has to offer the world.

Yoga, stemming from the Sanskrit meaning "union" or "yoke," is very closely related to the word *religion*. In Latin, *re* + *ligare* would translate to something akin to, "To tightly bind again." We get the word *ligament* from the same root. Bones are held tightly together with ligaments—it is a firm bond. *Yoga*, too, implies a uniting, a coming together in a lasting way. *Raja* ("royal") *yoga* is the term commonly given to sage Patañjali's teachings of the eight (*ashtangha*) branches of spiritual yoga. *Raja Yoga* and *Ashtangha Yoga* are interchangeable terms.

Unfortunately, many people know of yoga only as a series of physical stretches, but this is a gross misperception of the traditions from which yoga has emerged over millennia. Physical yoga, or *hatha yoga*, is but a small (although not insignificant) part of the holistic system of consciousness transformation that is yoga. The eight aspects, or "limbs," of Raja Yoga are these:

> *There are two kinds of yoga: hatha yoga and raja yoga. The hatha yogi practices physical exercises. Their goal is to acquire physical longevity and psychic abilities. But the aim of the raja yogi is the attainment of devotion, ecstatic love, knowledge and renunciation. Of these two, raja yoga is better.* Ramakrishna

- *Yamas*: five moral practices, restraints, which make you a beneficial and productive member of society, and which refine the ego.
- *Niyamas*: five behavioral practices, adherences, that start you on the road (and keep you prospering on the road) to transforming your consciousness and merging into the Higher Self.
- *Asana*: physical postures designed to tune up the endocrine, nervous, and musculoskeletal systems. The essential purpose of *asana* is to allow the aspirant to sit for extended periods in meditation and not get distracted by an uncomfortable body; greater strength and physical longevity are added benefits.
- *Pranayama*: harnessing vital energy through breathing exercises and awareness, primarily to magnetize the spinal column and increase the vitality reserve for more profound states of consciousness.
- *Pratyahara*: withdrawal or introspection of consciousness—prompting the aspirant to turn inward to uncover the ever-abiding holiness within.
- *Samyama—the collective actions of dharana, dhyana, and samadhi*: the last stages of attuning to God consciousness; the deeper, more advanced practice of turning inward, uniting mind with Spirit; the key components of the systematic progression toward enlightenment.

It is through these eight stages, each building on the practice of the one preceding it, that Patañjali and the readings' source delineate a course, a time-tested prescription, for transforming ego consciousness into Christ Consciousness and maximizing the valuable opportunity of an incarnation. This system brings you into an awareness of God where no fabricated dogma, institutional chastening, or metaphysical threats are involved or needed. This is an interesting coincidence of the readings and the yogic masters' teachings (one of numerous)—heaven and hell are what you make them to be—they are states of consciousness.

Transforming consciousness is the central focus in mysticism, the "inner" or "hidden" religious teachings found throughout every tradition. In spiritual yoga, even such ideas as past-life knowledge and telekinesis, although entertaining, are to be subservient to moral actions and daily, ever-deepening attunements to the Source.

> *Not all people, by any means, [who profess a belief in God, actually] believe in God. They simply talk. The worldly-minded people have heard something from someone that God exists and that everything happens by His will; but it is not their inner belief. Do you know what a worldly man's idea of God is like? It is like the children swearing by God when they quarrel. They have heard the word while listening to their elderly aunts quarrel.*
>
> *Ramakrishna*

Both the great teachers of Asian traditions, the lot of whom I will group together for the sake of efficiency as "sages" or "masters," and the Cayce readings' source have no patience for those of us who seek shortcuts. The readings' source states unambiguously that "there are no [short cuts] in Christianity" and "no short cuts to knowledge, to wisdom, to understanding," or to "spirituality." Everyone must pay the required price by working through the ego's foibles and rebellion—thought by thought, action by action. Fortunately, there is a well-traveled path in the yoga of the Christ. All we have to do is to commit to live it and work diligently for more inner Light.

Enlightenment is the natural result of taming the ever-sly ego and willfully surrendering to Spirit. It is not an easy task. Many of the skeptics, those who either completely discount all spiritual efforts as futile or those who think yoga is a threat to their belief system, are condemning the water as unpalatable before it reaches their own taste buds. They are misled by either fear or ignorance, both of which are perpetual roadblocks to spiritual awakening. But it is a choice, and everyone's reality is shaped by his or her choices.

Ultimately, spiritual yoga is a roadmap that charts the course for new choices, more expansive thoughts, and beneficial actions. It is a means to transform the seemingly intractable ways of the ego. The sages understood the ego's workings and knew that with knowledge comes responsibility. True knowledge, that which everyone seeks on the deepest level, is God knowledge—that which pulls the ego out of its narrow and troublesome confines, that which makes decisions not on sociopolitical or financial presumptions but on intuitive wisdom, that which is willing to sacrifice for the good of the whole.

The twenty-first century is ushering in a greater dialogue between spiritual knowledge and scientific curiosity. The experiences and wisdom of the ancient sages is interlocking with and helping to birth new discoveries in cellular biology, quantum physics, neuroplasticity, and mind-over-body protocols.

It is here, at this juncture, where spiritual yoga becomes a vital medicine. It is only by experiencing deeper states of consciousness that religion starts to make sense and has authentic meaning. It is only by delving into the nature of the mind, participating in the process of awakening, that scientists can know metaphysical reality as a fact of their own being. Then they can understand that there are certain things that can be measured and quantified . . . and other things, sacred things, which cannot.

This is how spiritual yoga can generate world peace—providing an opportunity for each individual to experience the sacred foundation upon which our very existence rests. Upon this understanding there can be no quarreling, no textual debate, and no sociopolitical factionalism. To put it in the vein of the sages: Once the inner light dawns, all the external darkness of argument and fear evaporates. This is but one of the priceless gifts of spiritual yoga for humanity.

1

The Yoga Sutras of Patañjali

There is virtually nothing historically reliable to help us know Patañjali. Patañjali may have been an individual spiritual adept or merely identified by a collection of writings, perhaps developed over centuries, attributed to one teacher. Regardless of this enigma, the Yoga Sutras reflect the culmination of a philosophical climax. These sutras weave together different philosophical elements and yet remain as a distinct composition able to defend itself against rival beliefs of the time, circa 200 C.E. One scholar believes them to be the fusion of two methodologies, kriya yoga and ashtangha yoga.[1]

The following is a reinterpretation of Patañjali's Yoga Sutras for the modern Western reader, especially in the light of the Edgar Cayce readings. It is not meant to be a direct translation as much a revitalized spiritual rendition faithful to the ethos and wisdom of the sutras.

These sutras should not be read in a hasty manner. They were originally meant to be discussion and instruction points between teacher and student. Keeping this in mind, each line and paragraph is a meditation in and of itself. Patañjali condensed profound mystical philosophies into small spaces. In reading these sutras, one should travel slowly and continually ask oneself, How does this apply to me? These words are not so much expositional as they are symbolic, meant to impel you to dive within the depths of your mind and heart.

Book I: On Concentration

This is the explanation of spiritual yoga:

Yoga is the prevention of the mind's constant agitation. In doing so, the seer eventually abides in the Self—the internal, boundless effulgence. When the mind is agitated, the seer erroneously identifies with mental agitations.

The mental agitations fall into five types, some of which are more problematic than others: ripe knowledge, unripe knowledge, the illusions of the intellect and imagination, dreams, and memory.

Ripe knowledge has three aspects: direct perception, sensible reasoning, and testimony from reliable sources.

Unripe knowledge is the development of an illusion based on misperception or misinformation. The illusion is mistaken for truth.

The illusion of the intellect is the assumption that scientific laws, theories, and postulations truly explain things as they are or that they have an enduring value. Concepts such as time, space, gravity, and so on, can only be understood in their effects, not in their meaning or value. The illusion of the imagination is like a pair of colored sunglasses (imagination) creating a fantastic, although misleading, panorama. There are some who do not effectively deal with reality because of the unrestrained trickery of their imagination. Superstitions, fears, neuroses, and the like, stem from this illusion.

Dreams are the storehouse of the conscious mind—the "schoolhouse" for the self. They reflect to the dreamer all that has been put into one's consciousness. They also make connections to higher realizations if consistent meditation and practice of the *yamas* and *niyamas* (the moral and ethical principles of spiritual yoga) are lived.

Memory, in this context, means the repetitive, mental reenactment of past events, the emotional clinging to mental impressions. It is a type of psycho-emotional antique collecting, and an agitation.

By spiritual practice and wisdom, these agitations can be transformed.

Spiritual practice is the repetition of activities that promote serenity and harmony in the body–mind. Meditation is the cornerstone of spiritual practice, eventually creating mental tranquility devoid of agitations. Spiritual practice must be consistent and imbued with fervid devotion for it to be a reliable foundation to Higher Mind.

Wisdom occurs as the result of the mind losing its fascination with the external, sensory world in favor of the internal luminescence—when the mind no longer depends on scriptures for spiritual understanding, when the mind is unencumbered by agitations. Wisdom gained through freedom of agitation is a kind of bliss—an embryonic bliss. This stage of embryonic bliss can also be cultivated through devoted faith and reverence, an increase in vital energy, perfect absorption in a sacred mantra, and one–pointed concentration upon, and union with, the Self—they all reinforce each other.

Spiritual aspirants with intense devotion and superior concentration achieve the greatest results in the shortest time. There are different methods and varying rates of intensity for particular seekers. Even among spiritual aspirants who share an intense devotion and practice a superior concentration, there will be differences in development.

Special devotion to the Christ Light helps facilitate spiritual transformation. The Christ Light is the supreme spiritual ideal; it is the infallible and genuine guru; it is the Light of the Higher Self. There is no limitation to its power; it is not constrained by time or space. The sacred word that attunes an aspirant to the Christ Light is AUM. Devotees repeat it and contemplate its true meaning by entering into its depth. In the AUM is revealed the Self from the ego self, the eternal from the transient, and the righteous from the inane. In the AUM is found spiritual insight and enduring wisdom.

There are numerous distractions to spiritual insight and enduring wisdom: physical or mental illness; incompetence, negligence; unresolved doubt, indecisiveness; perpetually delusive thinking, mistaken notions of enlightenment; slothfulness, idleness; no self–control; poor interpretation of the teachings, literalism; and unwillingness to consistently introspect and quiet the agitations. These are all significant impediments.

There is also mental residue, the previously mentioned mental antiques that cause problems. Depression, poor self-esteem, physical restlessness, and uneven or poor breathing (from an emotional import, not a physical anomaly) all arise from distractions that need to be rectified. Genetic disorders, biochemical imbalance, neglecting to resolve present-life troubles, and past-life patterns impressed upon the subconscious mind are among causal factors.

To rectify these impediments, single-pointed concentration should be learned and practiced regularly. This eventually leads to mental purification.

One can purify the mind through exercising kindness, charity, goodwill, and even-mindedness in all activities. This should be extended to all, especially those who emit the most negative of emotions. One can also purify the mind by learning *pranayama* (breathing exercises), concentrating on a transmundane idea, seeing deeply into the nature of things, discovering a mind that is free of agitations, taking dream images into meditation and meditation ideals into dreams, or by surrendering completely to the internal Christ Light. These all work if pursued in earnest.

When the mind is purified, the meditator, the process of meditation, and the object of meditation all fuse into one.

Ultimately, a nonduality consciousness is gained and oneness is directly perceived; words are no longer divorced from the things that they represent or symbolize. Also, memory impressions are cleansed, and things are perceived not through their associated memories but through direct, intuitive understanding of them. This type of intuitive understanding is fresh and unsullied by time and space.

At the superficial end of this intuitive continuum, experiences are transferable (to a degree) to logical thought and can be contained within structures of language. At the deeper end of this intuitive continuum, experiences are not transferable into logical thought and cannot be contained within structures of language. These are the two basic levels of spiritual intelligence.

This consciousness of nonduality transcends that which is found in texts, myths, fables, allegories, or testimonies. This unified consciousness is the result of consistent and devoted spiritual practice; it is the reward of skillful, spiritual yoga. At this stage the mind returns to infinite spaciousness, its original state, and the ego self begins to dissolve.

Book II: On Practice

Spiritual yoga is established by the practice of *tapas, svadhyaya,* and *Isvara-pranidhana* (explanation to follow). Spiritual yoga is a medicine for curing psycho-emotional afflictions; it is the foundation for creating enlightenment. There are five major afflictions: Ignorance (misconceiving the true nature of things), selfishness (ego worship), attachment (most often to pleasures), aversions (most often from vexations or discomforts), and the fear of death.

Ignorance is mistaking the corruptible for the pure, the imaginary for the absolute, the delusive for the truthful, and the ephemeral for the perennial. It clings to impurity, thinking it pure; misery, thinking it happiness; savagery, thinking it holy.

Selfishness is making a god of the ego and expecting everyone to willingly serve that false god, punishing those who do not.

Attachments are pleasure memories of the senses that one insists on recreating—they are unreal.

Aversions are psycho-emotional pain memories that one insists on not exposing to the Light—they are unreal.

The fear of death is an instigator of numerous neuroses for many people—there is no death, only an eviction of the spirit from its physical repository.

The five major afflictions are the root cause of the incarnational cycles. The incarnate Christ taught us not to put our energies into the things of this world, where moth and rust corrupt, because of the inherent afflictions possible in this realm. (Matthew 6:19) The five major afflictions are potential consequences of being born into the earth plane—all beings are feasibly subject to them.

One should be aware of one's attractions and aversions because they are a root cause of incarnations. One should be aware of one's attractions and aversions because they determine one's karmic trajectory. A sage is neither captured by attractions nor repulsed by aversions. However, even sages can be controlled by the ancient desire for self-preservation. Christ Consciousness is the perfect transcendence of the desire for self-preservation, gained through consistent and devoted spiritual practice.

Each of the five major afflictions has three levels: exoteric (sensory), esoteric (extrasensory), and etheric (spiritual). *Tapas* helps transform exoteric afflictions, *svadhyaya* assists in correcting esoteric afflictions, and *Isvara-pranidhana* recalibrates the nature of etheric afflictions.

These three levels of the five afflictions can be used as a means for personal liberation or further entrapment. Once you can distinguish the self from the Self, the liberating potential of sensory, extrasensory, and spiritual activity expands. Accomplishing this is an essential purpose of having an incarnation. Ignorance of the self from the Self, and the inability to use sensory, extrasensory, and spiritual means for liberation, is the mainspring of karmic suffering.

It is the perfect mastery over the three levels of the five afflictions—knowing the self from the Self; creating liberation via sensory, extrasensory, and spiritual means; and persistent consistency in the practice of *tapas, svadhyaya* and *Isvara-pranidhana*—that concepts such as "knowing God," enlightenment, *samadhi, nirvana,* or "spiritual liberation" are realized—fulfilling an individual entity's truest and deepest need.

At some point, perhaps after years or lifetimes of productive effort in spiritual yoga, one's thoughts, words, and actions fuse into a continuous, spiritual circuit. This leads to the obliteration of suffering. The continuous spiritual circuit has seven facets that must all be effectively integrated: spiritualized desires; purified attachments (attachment only to things which facilitate enlightenment); coalescence of body, mind, and spirit; realization of the Self; living one's highest ideal; metacognition; and attainment of mystical wisdom. Spiritual yoga facilitates their integration.

There is an eight-limbed process for attaining enlightenment through spiritual yoga. This process includes the practicing of the *yamas* (restraints), *niyamas* (adherences), *asanas* (physical postures), *pranayama* (breathing awareness), *pratyahara* (withdrawal), *dharana* (internalization), *dhyana* (meditation), and *samadhi* (spiritual bliss).

The five *yamas* are *ahimsa, satya, asteya, brahmacharya,* and *aparigraha.*
The five *niyamas* are *shauca, santosha, tapas, svadhyaya,* and *Isvara-pranidhana.*

The *yamas* and *niyamas* address the correction of perverse thoughts, which are the incessant causes of misery and perpetual ignorance.

As the spiritual aspirant develops immersion in *ahimsa* (nonviolence), all beings that come near will lose their hostile thoughts. As *satya* (truthfulness) is established, all that the aspirant says will manifest (according to God's laws.) As the aspirant lives *asteya* (nonstealing), all material things will manifest when needed. When *brahmacharya* (energetic conservation) is practiced, vital energy is increased and the aspirant then feels healthier and sharper mentally and has more vital energy to ascend through the spine for enlightenment. As *aparigraha* (noncovetousness) is faithfully abided by, knowledge of past lives is naturally revealed. When (*shauca*) purity of body and mind is sustained, psychosomatic well-being, healing, and virtue are increased as well as a greater potential for God realization. With the adherence to *santosha* (contentment) comes unlimited and unremitting joy. *Tapas,* or *tapasaya* (austerities), destroys impurities in the body–mind and helps alleviate negative karma. As *svadhyaya* (study of self and the sacred texts) is practiced, a greater discrimination is developed between the ego and the soul; the aspirant realizes the difference between the lower self and the higher Self. Unfathomable bliss is attained here on earth through constant surrender to the internal Lord (*Isvara-pranidhana.*)

Asanas (postures) should be motionless or facilitate a greater ease of motionless effort. As *asana* is perfected, meditation upon the Infinite should be increased. When done well, it expedites immunity toward all dualities of the world, for example, hot and cold, smooth and rough, easy and difficult, and so forth.

Once *asana* has been correctly established, *pranayama* (breath and vital energy control) is practiced. *Pranayama* has expansive, contractive, and retentive capacities. *Pranayama* should be performed with mindful control and attention to subtlety. There is a fourth type of *pranayama* that transcends the first three, but only by going through the first three. The veil covering enlightened mind can then be dissolved. (*Note: The fourth type of pranayama is intentionally not included here, as it is an advanced breathing technique not meant for public "intellectual consumption" but only for advanced adepts working closely with a God-realized teacher.)*

When the mind controls the externally directed habits of the senses, this is *pratyahara* (withdrawal.) As such, the mind becomes prepared for *dharana* (concentration.)

Book III: On Psychic Powers

Dharana (concentration) is the fixation of the mind on a particular holy idea. When *dharana* is perfected, the result is *dhyana* (meditation.) When self (ego) is lost in meditation, this is a type of "putting together," or *samadhi*.

Dharana, *dhyana*, and *samadhi* together are known as *samyama* (integration), and by mastering *samyama*, Christ Consciousness dawns. The benefits of *samyama* develop in stages. The transformations via *samyama* are subtle and profound.

Samyama addresses the *vrittis* (waves) of the conscious mind that breed spiritual ignorance via mental restlessness. Arresting thoughts before they arise and reveling in the bliss in between thoughts arising are parts of *samyama* practice. Leveling all impulsive thoughts is also part of the practice. Through the one-pointed absorption of *samyama*, many things can be known and revealed. In seeing the nature of the unseen (esoteric), the manifest (exoteric), and the potential to be (etheric), the various metaphysical strata can be known.

Knowledge of past and future lives can burgeon in *samyama*. One can know any word in any language, both the word itself and the thing it symbolizes, in *samyama*. Knowledge that other minds carry can be seen in *samyama*.

One can change one's physical form by entering the essence of perception. One can gain foreknowledge of one's physical death.

By applying *samyama* on virtues such as generosity, sympathy, and fellowship, a great strength and benevolence of the heart arises.

By applying *samyama* on physical strength, superhuman physical power can be developed.

By applying *samyama* to the inner light, things at a great distance can be seen and known.

By applying *samyama* to the solar plexus area, esoteric information regarding cosmic regions can be known. By applying *samyama* to the forehead region, esoteric information about astrogalaxies can be known.

By applying *samyama* to the hypogastric plexus, physiological structures can be seen and known.

By applying *samyama* to the throat (*vishuddha*) chakra, hunger and thirst can be controlled or eliminated.

By applying *samyama* to the nasopharyngeal area, great peace and calmness can be attained.

By applying *samyama* to the crown chakra, visions of the great masters can be had.

Samyama breeds intuitive cognition, and through intuitive cognition, everything can be known.

By applying *samyama* to the heart region, knowledge of the levels of consciousness can be known.

By applying *samyama* to the inner Light, extraordinary powers of hearing, touch, sight, taste, and smell can be cultivated.

Although the previously mentioned powers may seduce or coax the aspirant into chasing after them, know that they are all essentially distractions to *samadhi*, or Christ Consciousness.

The highest application of *samyama* is discrimination between self and Self, between ego shadow and Christ Light. Pursuing psychic powers for the sake of pageantry, flamboyance, vanity, or merchantry is an act of ego and an idea excoriated by the masters. These powers may arrive as the result of raising one's consciousness, but they are never to be clung to, coveted, or exploited. Masters encourage disciples not to attach to them and to move beyond them.

Book IV: On Liberation

Psychic powers can manifest as the result of several different actions: from incarnating (bringing them into a present life from past-life development), from ingesting specific herbs and plants, from repeating incantations transmitted from a God-realized master, from repetitive practice of a certain *tapas,* or from intense concentration.

Mental abilities should be used to remove obstacles to liberation, like a strong man that removes a dam, allowing the fields to be flooded.

All one's mental scaffolding exists as a result of individuality consciousness. There is only one Mind and millions of reflections of the one Mind.

We are often compelled by our subconscious mind because of the similarity between our karmic soul impressions and memories, both of which skirt the frontiers of the subconscious.

We have as a base desire a need for self-preservation, which is a kind of ancient default. This subliminal impression follows us life to life because it is lodged as a subconscious impression. If one can deconstruct the subconscious need for self-preservation, one can change the linkage of desires that keep one incarnating. This is one key aspect of Christ Consciousness. In this way *ahimsa* (nonviolence) becomes a natural extension of one's consciousness, along with the other *yamas* (explained further in the next chapter).

The many forms of reality are, in effect, the complex interplay between creation, sustenance, and destruction. All reality is, in some form, caught in the crosscurrents of these three principles.

External things have no reality of themselves, outside of a mind that perceives them. It is the perceiving mind that gives them a reality. Because of the Witness within—one's soul-level perception, a tiny extension of the Universal Mind—one can directly observe external things in their unreality as well as internal things as the true nature of the exoteric.

Each individual has a lower mind that can be observed by a Higher Mind. These are not two minds but two sides of one multiplex consciousness, separated by subliminal strata. The lower mind is called *manas*, and the higher mind is called *buddhi*, or pre-Christ Consciousness. Reprogramming *manas* and then transcending *manas* to *buddhi* are crucial steps to enlightenment.

For one who has realized the inner Christ Light as the Higher Mind, the Self, complex disciplines are unnecessary. For one who has not realized the inner Christ Light as the Higher Mind, the Self, complex disciplines are imperative in order to transform bad habits.

Our latent subliminal impressions will continue to affect our conscious decisions until we do this inner housecleaning.

After the full integration of the *yamas* and *niyamas* (moral/ethical principles of spiritual yoga), it is the refusal to engross oneself in the pursuit of psychic powers that leads to a higher opportunity—God realization. If *samyama* (integration of mind and spirit) is perfected and virtue cherished and maintained, mental agitations eventually cease, along with karma-producing actions. Then one's individuality is no longer under the control of the interplay between creation, sustenance, and destruction. In this way the individuality is "crucified," and all the elements holding together the idea of the physical body can disintegrate. This same disintegration will affect the mental body—then, eventually, the astral body. This is the advanced stage of enlightenment: At-one-ment, or God realization. Depending on how one chooses to perceive this process, it is a systematic disintegration of all mental and energetic habits that have created separation from the Source, or a systematic redirection of consciousness back to its holy Origin. This is authentic yoga.

2
Yamas: Rules for a Better World

In both the spiritual yogic systems of India and the teachings from the readings' source, one concept emerges as preeminent for spiritual development: Adherence to moral and ethical principles. There is no magic bullet or shortcut to God consciousness, only the steady transformation born of consistent and persistent spiritual practice. In the system of Raja ("royal") Yoga, the one systematized by Patañjali, the first and most critical stage of training for the spiritual aspirant is ethics/morals.

> Understood in the full sense of their meaning, [the yamas]² embrace the whole world of moral conduct. By their observance, the yogi avoids the primary or fundamental difficulties that could block his progress towards [God-consciousness.] Breaking the rules of moral conduct creates not only present misery, but long-lasting karmic effects that bind the devotee to suffering and mortal limitation.
>
> Paramahansa Yogananda

In Raja Yoga, the initial moral teachings are known as *yamas* ("observances"), a kind of thou–shalt–not–do set of rules for establishing optimal social harmony. Patañjali begins with these because he feels they transcend cultures and creeds. In the Yoga Sutras, he refers to them as "universal adherences." If everyone were to faithfully abide by these social rules, the world would be a much better, much safer, and more socially productive place.

15

The readings' source prompts everyone to seek Christ Consciousness as the highest spiritual choice. The recurring teaching in the readings is the need for the obliteration of "hate, prejudice, selfishness, backbiting, unkindness, anger, passion, and those things of the mire that are created in the activities of the sons of men." (5749–5) The sage Patañjali would be in full agreement with this formula. The following are the five *yamas*.

I. Ahimsa

First, do no harm.   Hippocratic Oath

Put your sword [away], for all who draw the sword will die by the sword.   Jesus; Matthew 26:52[3]

The Lord tests and proves the [unyieldingly] righteous, but [God's] soul abhors the wicked and him who loves violence.
                                                              Psalm 11:5

Thou shalt not kill.   Exodus 20:13 [King James Version]

Therefore all things whatsoever ye would that men should do to you, do ye even so to them . . .   Matthew 7:12 [KJV]

Love your enemies . . .   Jesus; Matthew 5:44 [KJV]

Father, forgive them, for they know not what they do.
                                                      Jesus; Luke 23:34

During a visit to the ashram of Mahatma Gandhi in 1935, I asked the prophet of nonviolence [ahimsa] for his definition of ahimsa. He replied: "The avoidance of harm to any living creature in thought or deed." A man of nonviolence neither willfully gives nor wishes harm to any. He is a paradigm of the golden rule: "Do unto others as you would have them do unto you."
                                                  Paramahansa Yogananda[4]

The first moral observance is *ahimsa*, meaning "nonharming" or perhaps "active nonviolence." This means not to purposefully

> There is no virtue higher than *ahimsa*.   Swami Vivekananda

harm anyone or anything or to live with the sincere intention of such. Intention is the key principle here, as it is impossible to wash one's hands or brush one's teeth without "harming" countless bacteria in the process. We have to be reasonable and pragmatic in the application of *ahimsa*.

In most of the Asian systems, degrees of efficacy are acknowledged as unavoidable in the practice of spiritual ideals. For example, if your family were about to be harmed by a person with criminal intent and you injured or fatally wounded the criminal in the process of protecting your family, this is not considered a violation of *ahimsa*. It is only when a person intends to harm another, and especially if that person enjoys it, that violating the moral of *ahimsa* is the cause for creating negative karma and adding to the collective pool of world suffering.

If, for example, in the course of a building project, you inadvertently knock down an inhabited bird's nest, this is not considered some grievous offense, especially if you take appropriate actions to restore it or move it to a safer location. Making mistakes should not be interpreted as an unpardonable wrongdoing—not learning from them or being apathetic toward them is the real problem. It is having the *intention* of nonharming that is most essential to living *ahimsa*. This would include consistently living with the awareness of reconciliation and forgiveness.

The readings' source implied on a few occasions or stated outright that the cause of physical ailments of numerous people seeking Mr. Cayce's counsel was their ridiculing or belittling others in past lives. This unmindful cruelty creates a *vikarma* (negative karma) that may take multiple lifetimes to eradicate. It also can create a *vikarma* that attracts ridicule and belittlement to one's self, now or later.

Besides creating harmonious relationships, adding to world peace, and insulating us from negative physical karma, an added benefit that faithfully adhering to *ahimsa* offers is a peaceful security that precedes us wherever we go. It is said that not even the wildest of beasts will harm a spiritual aspirant who faithfully lives *ahimsa*.

Ahimsa was the foundation for Gandhi's monumental social transformation in India. Martin Luther King Jr. was so taken with the idea, through Gandhi's example, that he and his associates visited India to learn more of *ahimsa* from Gandhi's protégées. Even the current Dalai Lama is a wonderful representative of the power of *ahimsa* when he refers to the Communist Chinese military, which forced him into exile and systematically decimated the Tibetans' country and culture, as "my greatest teachers." There is no call for revenge or a mandate for war, but instead he insists on education, peaceful activism, and patient noncompliance with his "teachers."

Jesus said he could have had "more than twelve legions of angels" to assist him in defeating his enemies (Matthew 26:53), yet he chose forgiveness and sacrifice. He, too, lived *ahimsa*.

There are some who adhere to a vegan diet, thinking that that alone is the supreme embodiment of *ahimsa*. From the standpoint of many of the masters, it is not what goes into one's

[L]ongsuffering . . . does not mean suffering of self and not grumbling about it. Rather, though you [are] persecuted, unkindly spoken of, taken advantage of by others, you do not attempt to fight back or to do spiteful things; [non-violence means] that you be patient—first with self, then with others.   3121-1

mouth that counts as much as what comes out of it (words and deeds). One may be vegan and still be plagued with neuroses of jealousy, envy, pridefulness, and materialism. The following quote is but one example of a recurring teaching:

> The test of *ahimsa* is absence of jealousy. Any man may do a good deed, or make a good gift on the spur of the moment or under the pressure of some superstition of priestcraft; but the real lover of mankind is he who is jealous of none. The so-called "great men of the world" are seen to become jealous of each other for a small name, for a little fame, and for a few bits of gold. So long as this jealousy exists in a heart, it is far away from the perfection of *ahimsa* . . . Any fool may abstain from

eating this or that; surely that gives him no more distinction than the herbivorous animals. The man who will mercilessly cheat widows and orphans, and do the vilest things for money, is worse than any brute, even if he lives entirely on grass. The man whose heart never cherishes even the thought of injury to another, who rejoices at the prosperity of even his greatest enemy—that man is a *bhakta* (a devotee of God's love), he is a [true] yogi, [and] he is the guru of all, even though he lives every day of his life on the flesh of swine.   Swami Vivekananda[5]

The *ahimsa* concept recurs consistently in the teachings of the masters. Perhaps, one day enough people will be thoroughly convinced and motivated to actualize it. Then we will see the dawn of a new planet. What is most important is for us to implement it in all we do. *Ahimsa* is the foundation upon which all the *yamas* and *niyamas* are built.

II. Satya

If you abide in My Word [*logos*, Christ Consciousness] . . . you are truly My disciples. And you will know the truth, and the truth will set you free. Jesus; John 8:31-32 [KJV; author's brackets]

Blessed are the pure in heart: for they shall see God.
Jesus; Matthew 5:8 [KJV]

Those who are in that way or attitude of "Let the words of my mouth and the meditation of the heart be acceptable in Thy sight," are in the way of truth.   262-77

In breaking through from those things that hinder in the material, such as would defile the body, numb the senses or make for impurities in the body, *from* such abstain. In those that make for love, purity of purpose, of aim, these bring the light of the glory of the Father, who so loved us as to give His Son. In this manner, then, may the will, the call, the understanding, come to thine *own* self . . .   294-139

[Satya] is the foundation stone of the universe . . . Men and civilizations stand or fall according to their attitude toward truth.

Paramahansa Yogananda[6]

Satya means to be truthful with your words and actions. It does not allow any room for deception, duplicity, or psychological manipulation bolstered by guile or falsehood. This is a high

One does not spiritually succeed as long as they have these three: shame, hatred, and fear.

Sri Ramakrishna

ideal, but the readings' source stipulates in numerous ways that man's ways and God's ways are seldom the same. We *need* high ideals in order to awaken spiritually. A deep understanding of this breeds *satya*.

It is a firm verbal and ideological commitment to truthfulness that gives one's words the power to manifest a new reality, to create what is needed. It is not merely visualizing that manifests something, it is the quality of consciousness of the seeker. If our internal "dial" is tuned to God consciousness, we are better able to manifest what we need, as our needs naturally become simplified and in accord with the Divine plan; we then have the intuitive discrimination to know what is acceptable and unacceptable in the big picture and the will to realize it.

Mahatma Gandhi made the bedrock of his philosophy the first two *yamas—ahimsa* and *satya—* which he termed *satyagraha*. Look at what he accomplished by giving 100 percent to only two of the

An ideal . . . *cannot, should* not, *will* not, be that that is man-made, but must be of the spiritual nature—that has its foundation in Truth, in God . . .

262-11

ten transformational precepts! As he committed to making them foremost in his personal philosophy, countless others were, and still are, affected by that commitment. This is why the sages declare that the *yamas* and *niyamas* have powerful personal and global transformative potential, but only to the degree that we faithfully live them. It can be difficult, but we must not give up on ourselves or one another. What is exponentially more difficult is a life ungoverned by spiritual precepts.

Ultimately, *satya* means to live in line with "eternal truth." There are three basic levels to *satya*:

1. Conscious satya—in which the logical mind finds truthful corroborations in philosophy and other manmade schemes. These relate to many ethical and moral principles to "be honest," "tell the truth," and the like. These are important.

2. Subconscious satya—in which the truths are presented in dream visions and intuitive messages. These are sublime.

3. Superconscious satya—in which the truths presented to the seeker come in visions and "paranormal" experiences. These are commonly referred to as "mystical experiences," and though erroneously labeled as "paranormal," they are of the most natural manifestations of spiritual awakening.

The ideal intention of *satya* is to live purity in word and action. To speak one's "truth" under the guise of cruelty, malice, or malevolence is not *satya* but a type of ego-induced blindness. One

> *So few in this world discriminate properly between their want and their need.*   Hazrat Inayat Khan

must be truthful while being compassionate, honoring the initial teaching of *ahimsa*. If you cannot speak your truth and be compassionate, wait to speak until you can. You cannot honor *satya* and simultaneously defy *ahimsa*. It does not matter that the "truth" is accurate—if it is conveyed in a malevolent and hurtful manner, it is antithetical to both *ahimsa* and *satya*. We all have a responsibility to speak the truth in a compassionate manner if we are to honor the spirit of *satya* and the *yamas* as a whole. If we can stay faithful to this, the power of our words can manifest great things.

III. Asteya

The thief comes only in order that he may steal and may kill and

> may destroy. I came that they may have and enjoy life, and have
> it in abundance . . .   Jesus; John 10:10

> In its most covetous and avaricious display, greed leads to steal-
> ing, dishonesty, cheating, self-surfeit at the expense of the well-
> being of others. If man allows himself to be conquered by greed,
> his life and spirit will be ruined and shattered by suffering.
> Paramahansa Yogananda[7]

Asteya is the yogic version of the biblical commandment "Thou shalt not steal." It means not to *want* to steal from another, as much as refraining from the act itself.

It is thought in the yogic traditions that adherence to *asteya* eventually brings remembrance of one's past lives. It seems that a large part of past lives being blocked from our conscious mind is the result of our greedy nature—not only materialism, but clinging to the present life.

IV. Brahmacharya

> [F]or I have betrothed you to one Husband, to present you as a
> chaste virgin to Christ. But [now] I am fearful lest that even as
> the serpent beguiled Eve by his cunning, so your minds may be
> corrupted and seduced from wholehearted . . . and pure devo-
> tion to Christ [Consciousness].
> Paul of Tarsus; 2 Corinthians 11:2-3 [author's brackets]

> Man is man so long as he is struggling to rise above nature—
> and this nature is both internal and external . . . it is good and
> very grand to conquer external nature, but grander still to con-
> quer our internal nature. It is grand and good to know the laws
> that govern the stars and planets; it is infinitely grander and
> better to know the laws that govern the passions, the feelings,
> and the will, of mankind.   Swami Vivekananda[8]

The word *Brahmacharya* translates as "knower of Brahma," or one who knows Eternal Spirit, and the concept means practicing sexual moderation as a key principle to raising sacred, spiritual energies from the lower spinal centers to the higher ones.

Not everyone is called to celibacy, and for some, the readings'
source counseled, celibacy would
be disastrous. It is more an issue
of how to transform energy than
repress it. *Brahmacharya* is the
process of transforming sexual

Chastity in thought, word and deed always and in all conditions, is called brahmacharya.
        Swami Vivekananda

energies into spiritual magnetism, most notably in the spine. This magnetism eventually rises into the brain for higher states of spiritual realization.

Both the readings' source and the great Eastern masters recommend moderation of sexual activity and, ultimately, transformation of it. The Cayce readings counseled people to "*subdue* the influences [forces] of materiality" (1056-2), noting that "from the desires of the heart do the activities of the brain, of the physical being, shape that [which you would create]" (276-3). [author's brackets]

Sexual energy is a powerful, creative force, perhaps humans' most powerful physical energy. If this energy is sublimated and raised to the higher spiritual centers, the deeper and more sublime states of God consciousness can be realized.

Both the masters and the readings' source call on all spiritual aspirants to take inventory of their desires:

> [T]hat which is carnal and that which is mental and that which is spiritual may be found—in *desire*. For [desire] builds—and is that which is the basis of evolution, and of life [procreation], and of truth. . . It also takes hold on hell and paves the way for many that find themselves oft therein.   262-60

The masters also counsel couples in the art of spiritualized living, teaching that mutual respect and honor are destroyed by reckless and self-indulgent sexual activities:

> Husbands and wives who think that the "holy bonds of matri-
> mony" permit them to indulge in oversexuality, greed, anger, or
> displays of "temperament" are ignorant of the true laws of life.
> The [growing numbers] of inharmonious families and the rising
> number of divorces found everywhere today are glaring warn-
> ings that marriage does not mean license to indulge the de-
> sires, lusts, moods, and emotions of the senses.
>
> Paramahansa Yogananda[9]

Sexual desire is addressed in the *yama* of *brahmacharya*, but truthfully, all the *yamas* and *niyamas* address desire in one form or another—the desire to retaliate with violence (*ahimsa*), the desire to steal (*asteya*), and so on. The key point for those wanting to incorporate these principles into their lives is not to aspire to perfect desirelessness, to stagger around in an apathetic, comatose state, but to spiritualize desires, so that they become fuel for the purest desire of Christ Consciousness and universal love. As opposed to suppressing desires, spiritualizing desires is the rec-ommended method in the readings.

The great Bengali saint Sri Ramakrishna is often quoted as saying that "women and gold," or lust and greed, are the major obstacles to God consciousness. Cayce said, "*Nothing* may separate the soul of man from its Maker but desires and lusts." (1293–1) In our current era, in which some are misguided into supposed tantric practices, deluded into thinking there is something spiritual about amusing themselves with sexual theatrics, it is wise to recall the teachings of the masters and the readings' source. The astute person remains unconvinced by a heroin addict's argument that narcotic–filled needles are not at all dangerous, despite the junkie's elaborate sales pitch and professionally produced DVD "The Ecstatic Joys of Heroin."

An entire chapter, Lesson IV, is dedicated to desire in *A Search for God*, Book II. Here Cayce and his close associates who helped de-velop the book's materials ad-dress desire on many levels.

From what may *anyone* be saved? Only from themselves! That is, their indi-vidual hell; they dig it with their own desires!   262-40

Desire is presented as an act of will, and all that we attract to ourselves is relative to the desires that we hold. The carnal, or lower three,
chakra energies of "self-preservation, propagation of the species, and
hunger" are presented in the readings as "primary urges," which are
often used for "self-aggrandizement," or expansion of the ego. It is clearly
stated that "physical desires which are not spiritualized hinder the development of the consciousness of oneness with God."

This is in perfect accord with the spiritual masters, who counsel the
need to refine desires and convert carnal appetites into a higher vibrational level through devoted spiritual practice.

Since one of humanity's oldest physical desires is lust, *brahmacharya*
addresses this dilemma by advocating sexual moderation and, where
appropriate, chastity. The next part of understanding *brahmacharya* is
learning how to reperceive sexuality as an expression of the mind's
need to create. Once the aspirant realizes that sexuality does not have
to be externally expressed but can be redirected internally as fuel for
cultivation of enlightened mind, the doors to higher perceptions can
open with time and patience. After all, 99 percent of our experience of
the world, including sex, is mental.

Surrendering to lust, the mahayogis warn, has manifold consequences: moodiness, depression, irritability, and a gradual weakening
of the immune system—all manifestations of vital force depletion in the
body and energies being imprisoned in the lower, carnal centers. Living
in those lower centers eventually weakens you on numerous levels.

In the yogic traditions, celibacy is considered the ideal for the unmarried and elderly. For married couples, sexual enjoyment is not supposed to usurp the deeper values of true friendship and committed
monogamous love. If one engages in sex as rote, an obligation, or mere
entertainment, the sacredness is stripped away and negative karma will
eventually poison the relationship. One can observe the effects of this
with many "marriages" that were just material procurements or arrange-
ments of sexual convenience. The American divorce rate, in excess of 60
percent, is a testimony to this, and there are other countries whose
marriage failure rate is even higher. We are "liberated" through indulg-
ing our whims and impulses, and it is not bringing us real happiness.

If the aspirant becomes aware enough to catch him– or herself losing moral high ground in relation to *brahmacharya*, there is a recipe to follow to rescue lost virtue. These are all reinforcing of one another and can be implemented in any order:

1. Keep your mind on holy, spiritualized thoughts and ideas. Focus on sacred passages in any of the revered religious texts.
2. Engage yourself in creative projects: writing, painting, music, or any creative endeavor that can be a productive channel for redirecting the energies.
3. Perform physical exercise while keeping your mind on some spiritually beneficial idea.
4. Hold to a vegetarian diet. Meats and many dairy foods (except ghee) are thought to contain animal vibrations that energetically influence you toward animal (lower vibrational) behaviors. Even if you practice vegetarianism for a limited time, it can be helpful.
5. Enjoy the frequent company of spiritual–minded associates and teachers.
6. Avoid all entertainment that exploits sexual ideas (music, movies, TV, Internet, books, etc.). If you have it in your dwelling, discard it.
7. Volunteer in a service capacity. Helping keep others healthy, sheltered, and well fed gets you out of that little egoistic drama. It is a wonderful experience to feel the freedom of service, and an effective activity to help unfetter the ego from neuroses.

The key point to remember with regard to *brahmacharya* is that it is not forced celibacy. Instead, it is seeing the Divine in the other, treating sex as a sacrament, knowing how and when to

> *To express an impulse gives relief, but to control it gives strength.*
> Hazrat Inayat Khan

practice restraint, and not abusing the physical act through depravity or excess.

If we cannot control our physical urges, no matter what they are, we are not putting enough commitment into living the spiritual precepts.

We are spiritual beings endowed with infinite creative power—we are not mere biological machines.

Since many teachers and systems have contributed to the yogic systems, there are multiple formulas that have been recommended throughout the centuries. Another ancient formula for adhering to *brahmacharya* can be shown in this five-point format:

1. Avoid all lusts (not just sexual ones).
2. Discipline your mind (*tapas*).
3. Keep to a pure, moderate diet and avoid all intoxicants (*shauca*).
4. Do not oversleep, as it dulls the mind and acts as a type of mental intoxicant.
5. Meditate daily and increase the depth of your attunement.

The following are some excerpts from the readings. Many people came to Mr. Cayce with relationship troubles of various kinds. The readings' source often gave advice similar to the Eastern masters, or at least in accord with the spirit of the *yamas* and *niyamas*.

(Q) How should love and the sexual life properly function?
(A) [T]he material things (or those in a three-dimensional world) are the shadow or the reflection of those in the spiritual life. Then, as God or the Creative Influence is the source of all things, the second law in spiritual life, in mental life, in material life, is preservation of self and the continuation . . . or propagation [of the species], in sexual intercourse or life.

Hence in their very basic forces, [sexual relations] should be the outcome—not the purpose of . . . the answering of soul to soul in their associations and relations. And the [sexual] act . . . should be the result.

Hence these questions should be often weighed well, remembering that God, or Love (for it is One), [looks] on the heart rather than the outward appearances. And that morality, virtue, understanding, truth, love, are those influences that make for [proper] judgments of . . . the material life . . . according to

those rules that govern such relationships, then it behooves—
and becomes necessary—that there be the adherence to such
[moral] regulations, that thy good be not [evilly] spoken of . . .

[K]now that Love and God are One; that relations in the sexual
life are the manifestations [of the creative power of mind].

For, unless [sexual] associations become [regulated by love
and physical moderation], they become vile in the experience of
those that join in such relations.   272-7

The readings implied on a few occasions that sexual activity between
two people, if engaged in for purely carnal reasons and without a true
heart connection, could produce offspring with physical and emotional
problems:

For, to be sure, relationships in the sex are the exercising of the
highest emotions in which a physical body may indulge. And
only in man is there found that such are used as that of *destruction* to the body-offspring!   826-6

The readings' source counseled numerous couples that sex is not just
for the act of creating a child but is the physical expression of spiritual
and emotional bonds:

(Q) So much has been written about sexual relationships between husband and
wife. Is it the correct understanding that this activity
should be used only and
when companions seek to
build a body for an incoming
entity?

Do not look upon sex as merely a
physical expression! There is a physical expression that is beauty within
itself, if it is considered from that angle;
but when the mental and the spiritual
are guiding, then the outlet for beauty
becomes a *normal* expression of a
normal, healthy body.   1436-1

(A) Not necessarily. These depend, of course, to be sure, on the
individual concept of relationships and their activities . . . [I]f the
activities are used in creative, spiritual form, there is the less

desire for carnal relationship; or, if there is the lack of use of constructive energies, then there is the desire for more of the carnal, physical reaction.   2072-16

The masters teach that we are here on earth not merely to pursue pleasure but to gain wisdom. The sages gain perfect control over their appetites, severing the carnal bonds that perpetuate reincarnation. If we learn how to transform sexual impulses into spiritual fuel, we can ascend in consciousness sooner rather than later.

Man may not live by bread alone. Man may not live by the gratifying of appetites in the material world. For man is not made for this world alone. There is a longing for those experiences which the soul . . . has experienced. And without spirituality the earth is indeed a hell, an individual soul do what it will or may. Such longing may not be gratified from without [externally] or in the . . . experiences that pertain to, the forces and influences without [outside of] self. For the body is indeed the temple of the living God. Act like it! Keep it clean. Don't desecrate it ever, but keep it such that it may be the place where you would meet [your] own better self, [your] own God-self. As [you] do this, there may be brought harmony, peace, joy. As in everything else, if [you] would have joy [you] must make others happy! Bring joy to others. If [you] would have love, [you] must show [yourself] lovely! If [you] would have friends, show [yourself] friendly! If [you] would know God, search for Him, for He is within [your] own self! And as [you] express Him in the fruits of spirit; love, grace, mercy, peace, longsuffering, patience, kindness, gentleness; [you] will find such within [yourself] . . . This is the source of life, the source of love, the source of peace, the source of harmony, and as [you] give expression to same, it may come indeed to [you].   4082-1

V. Aparigraha:

> Watch and be on your guard against avarice of any kind, for life does not consist in possessions, even when someone has more than he needs.   Jesus; Luke 12:15 [author's paraphrase]

> You bemoan not having what others have. You don't know what it is to be free. The contrast of the happiness within your soul outbalances all the pleasure that you can get from your senses. So don't spend too much time seeking and caring for possessions.   Paramahansa Yogananda[10]

Aparigrana means "nonavarice" and recommends keeping to a simple life. It is the old adage not to let your possessions possess you. This teaching is especially poignant in countries that have abundant material resources. This *yama* entreats us to "simplify, simplify, simplify," in the words of Thoreau, keeping our material needs to a minimum and our spiritual connection at full depth.

> Do not gather . . . and store for yourselves treasures on earth, where moth and rust and worm consume and destroy, and where thieves break through and steal; But gather . . . and store for yourselves treasures in heaven [God consciousness], where neither moth nor rust nor worm consume and destroy, and where thieves do not break through and steal.   Matthew 6:19-20

Since the post–World War I era, America has been on a track of progressive, some might contend reckless, consumption. We are now seeing the various effects of our excessive appetites in social and environmental imbalances. Other countries, in an attempt to keep up with the Joneses, are mimicking this behavior and reaping the detriments. If *aparigraha* were to be applied personally and globally, these present imbalances could be soon rectified. It is a precept that needs implementation in the wealthiest countries. However, we should all start with ourselves first—wherever we live.

3

Niyamas: Guidelines for Effective Self-Transformation

In the next series of yogic teachings, the adherences (*niyamas*) are pre-sented for the aspirant to incorporate. After integrating the rules for psychosocial propriety (*yamas*), one then works on transforming one's ego by faithful dedication to these following five tenets.

I. Shauca:

First clean the inside of the cup and of the plate, so that the outside may be clean also.   Jesus; Matthew 23:26

[L]et us cleanse ourselves from everything that contaminates and defiles body and spirit, and bring [our] consecration to com-pleteness in the [reverence] of God.
       Paul; 2 Corinthians 7:1 [final brackets author's]

[P]urity of purpose, of mind, of body, must be kept if there would be the mental or the spiritual urge that will bring peace and harmony in the experience in this sojourn.   259-8

[I]n entering into the silence . . . in meditation, with a clean hand, a clean body, a clean mind, we may receive that strength

and power that fits each individual, each soul, for a greater
activity in this material world.   281-13

As the body-physical is purified, as the mental body is made
wholly at-one with purification or purity, with the life and light
within itself, healing comes, strength comes, power comes.
                                                          281-24

Be spotless within. Make your inner self a temple of God.
                                   Paramahansa Yogananda[11]

One who is physically clean and is also rid of the mental taints
of uncontrollable desires and restless thoughts indeed invites
the Lord to manifest Himself in the purified temple of his life.
                                   Paramahansa Yogananda[12]

Shauca means "cleanliness" and includes both external and internal
cleansings.

External *shauca* consists of physical cleanliness in proper hygiene,
foods devoid of chemicals and synthetic processing, vegetarian diets,
therapeutic baths, refraining from alcohol or drug use, *hatha yoga* (physical) *asanas*, massage therapy, and medicinal herbal or botanical treatments. For external or physical *shauca*, colon hydrotherapy, sweating,
vigorous exercise and breathing, and cleansing foods are also commonly recommended in various wellness traditions. Common–sense
fasting, too, is a common *shauca*. (Refer to *The Alkalizing Diet*, chapter ten,
"The Seven Types of Fasts.")

Internal *shauca* consists of avoiding negative, destructive emotions:
arrogance, pride, conceit, malice, vengefulness, greed, lust, anger, de-
spair, and apathy are among the most commonly noted. All of these are
symptoms of the disease of spiritual rebellion. This emotional pollution
is a considerable roadblock to spiritual awareness.

The yogic masters put forth their version of *cleanliness is next to godli-
ness*, but not to a neurotic extreme. Many religions require cleansing
with water as a precursor to prayer or as an important symbolic ritual.

What is paramount as a regular part of psychospiritual attunement is to cleanse the mind of negative thoughts and images. This helps reinforce the benefits of consistent meditation. Besides being a sensible and beneficial public health protocol, *shauca* is required to increase one's spiritual vibration. In the spiritual yogic traditions, *shauca* is critical for proper development in the beginning and intermediate stages for all aspirants.

The masters prioritize inner cleanliness over the external, but common sense would dictate incorporating both.

In Mark's Gospel, Jesus dispossesses a young boy of an "unclean spirit," whereas the disciples could not:

> And when He had gone indoors His disciples asked him privately, Why could not we drive it out?
> And He replied to them, This kind cannot be driven out by anything but prayer and fasting.   Mark 9:28-29

The combination of prayer (attunement) and fasting (*shauca*) is a frequently employed combination in many spiritual cultures. This should empower the aspirant to rely less on physical means and more on spiritual ones.

[P]urity of purpose, of mind, of body, must be kept if there would be the mental or the spiritual urge that will bring peace and harmony in the experience in this sojourn.   259-8

II. Santosha

> Let your character . . . be free from love of money—[including] greed, avarice, lust, and craving for earthly possessions—and be satisfied with your present [circumstances . . .]; for He (God) . . . has said, "I will not in any way fail you . . . nor leave you without support . . . nor forsake nor let [you] down . . . "
> Hebrews 13:5

[I]n the meeting of karmic forces in each experience—then there

may be [built] that as will bring about . . . contentment which
makes for a life much worth while.   369-9

The idea of *santosha* is quite simple: accept whatever is in your life
right now as (1) the result of your actions, (2) the quality of your consciousness, and (3) the perfect circumstances to awaken Divine Mind.
This *niyama* prompts aspirants to accept the reality that *they* are responsible for their progress or lack thereof. *Santosha* allows no room for a
blind fatalism but instead states that everything that is in your life is
there for a reason—and *you* are that reason.

If you want roses and have none, start planting rose bushes now. If it
is blueberries that you lack, get busy planting those seeds, and in time,
the harvest is yours. The key idea is that we cannot blame anyone else
or anything for our life situation, not the boogeyman, not the devil, not
"bad luck," not the past, and especially not God. We have the divine gifts
of willpower and creativity in our minds and should consistently exercise them for positive, productive results. This is how the *yamas* and
niyamas empower the aspirant, and *santosha* is a key ingredient.

The readings' version of *santosha* can be summed up by the following:

"By applying what we know day by day" we gain a better understanding of ourselves and our spiritual knowledge.
                                           A Search for God, Book I

While there are those karmic influences that must be met, because of that which has been [built] by an entity . . . it must of
itself meet that which is the measure according to . . . universal
[law]. Or, to put it in another manner:
    It is not all for an entity, or a soul, to have knowledge con-
cerning law; whether karmic law, spiritual law, penal law, social
law, or what not. The *condition* [stipulation] is, what does the
entity *do about* the knowledge that is gained! Is the knowledge
used to evade cause and effect, or is it used to coerce individuals into adhering to the thoughts of self? or is it used to *aid*

others in *their* understanding *of* the law, and *thus* bring the
cause to that position where the will of the Creative influence is
supreme; or the power that comes with making the will one [in
harmony] *with* the law of love, of karma, of cause and effect, of
every influence—one *with* Creation!   342-2

Thus, by using our willpower wisely, we receive the grace of becoming one with the Creative Forces, or God.

III. Tapas (Tapasaya)

I have come to cast fire upon the earth, and how I wish that it
were already kindled!   Jesus; Luke 12:49

Whoever does not persevere and carry his own cross and come
after (follow) Me, cannot be My disciple.
    For which of you, wishing to build a farm-building, does not
first sit down and calculate the cost, whether he has sufficient
means to finish it?
    Otherwise, when he has laid the foundation and is unable to
complete [the building], all who will see it begin to mock and
jeer at him,
    Saying, This man began to build, and was not able (worth
enough) to finish.   Jesus; Luke 14:27-30

[I]n suffering, *strength* is gained . . .   5528-1

If there is any harmful habit that you have not yet tamed, learn
now to control it.   Paramahansa Yogananda[13]

Tapas means "heat" and is commonly translated to indicate "austerity" or "discipline." The point of *tapas* is to discover a deep joy and happiness that comes from conquering the whims, follies, and impulses of the body–mind. If discipline is implemented and no joy and happiness eventually emerge from one's efforts, the methods are faulty and need to be altered. In other words, *tapas* should not be used as a kind of justified violence to the body but as a method toward self–empowerment via ego transcendence.

Being patient and levelheaded under duress is a kind of *tapas*. Those who are upset easily by small sufferings, inconveniences, or annoyances are considered spiritually immature by both the readings' source and the mahayogis. In the Search for God lesson on patience, it is stated, "Patience is a virtue that has no vacation." The readings' source also returns numerous times to the idea that we live in the three dimensions of time, space, and patience. Patience, when it is correctly understood, perceives life events from a soul view and not an ego view, the latter of which is impatient and cannot see the big picture. *Tapas* helps move our consciousness into this soul–view outlook.

Force self to do some unpleasant things that it hasn't wanted to do once in a while, and like it!   911-3

Tapas has many facets. Keeping an even mental attitude in the midst of emotional turmoil or physical hardship and purposefully enduring challenging or uncomfortable things have been a part of the development of all religious traditions in one form or another. In addition, *tapas* includes the following:

1. Sexual conservation (*brahmacharya*)
2. Fasting and special diets
3. Physical activities and exercises designed to strengthen the body and mind
4. Patiently enduring heat, cold, and other environmental discomforts
5. Observing silence for extended periods of time
6. Advancing in stages through progressively challenging *asanas*
7. Eliminating idle talk (gossip, etc.) and curse words
8. Meditating for extended periods of time

True *tapas* helps us transcend ego–created confines and expand our mind–body potential. The extreme approach of some conservative religions (for example, "the body is bad and must be punished or considered to be 'evil'") on the one hand and that of many New Age sects (for example, "the body is intoxicating and should be worshiped, adored, and constantly doted on") on the other are both erroneous choices. The body is a divine vehicle, but merely a vehicle. The mind rules the body, and insufficient emphasis is placed on this in our culture. *Tapas* is pragmatic training to accomplish a greater awareness of spiritual empowerment via ego transcendence.

> Self-discipline is different from self-torture. The aim of *tapas* is not served by startling exhibitions, such as "fakirs" on beds of sharp nails. The profound purpose of *tapas* is to change in man his "bad taste" in preferring transient sense pleasures to the ever-lasting bliss of the soul. Some form of self-discipline is necessary to transmute material desires into spiritual aspirations. By tapas and meditation the devotee gives himself a standard of comparison between the two kinds of pleasures: physical and mental on one hand, and spiritual on the other.
>
> Paramahansa Yogananda[14]

The venerated teacher Swami Vivekananda says, *tapas* is

> a kind of penance to "heat" the higher nature. It is sometimes [implemented] in the form of a sunrise to sunset vow, such as repeating OM all day incessantly. Such a discipline produces a certain power that you can convert into any form you wish, spiritual or material . . . The Hindus even say that God practiced Tapas to create the world.[15]

Once again, we must be clear that the attachment to a physical exercise or regiment is not the goal of this *niyama*. *Tapas* is a purposeful exertion to expand our consciousness, not to create more somatic attachment. Yogananda clarifies the point:

> The ascetic who is busy with disciplining the body, putting it

through rigorous austerities, may attain a degree of control over the physical instrumentality; but merely practicing postures [asanas], enduring cold and heat, and not giving in to sorrow and pleasure—without simultaneously concentrating on Cosmic Consciousness—is only a roundabout pathway to gaining the mental control necessary for God-communion . . . Many devotees are so engrossed in following the precepts of external asceticism and renunciation that they forget that ecstasy with the Infinite is the purpose of such self-discipline.

Paramahansa Yogananda[16]

We must learn control over the body–mind but for the sole purpose of directing our attention wholly upon God.

IV. Svadhyaya

Seek first God's kingdom within, and all the things you need shall be given to you.

Jesus; Matthew 6:33 and Luke 12:31 [author's paraphrase]

First [know] self—for in knowing self one finds God. Keep thy paths straight.   97-2

The Self is your own nature . . . you are not to become pure, you are already pure. You are not to become perfect; you are already that. Nature is like a screen which is hiding the reality beyond. Every good thought you think or act upon tears the veil, as it were, and the Purity, the Infinity, the God behind, is manifested more and more . . . Finer and finer becomes the veil, more and more of the light behind shines forth; for it is its nature to shine.   Swami Vivekananda[17]

Search for the source of the "I"-thought. That is all that one has to do. The universe exists on account of the "I"-thought. If that ends there is an end to misery also. The false "I" will end only when its source is sought.   Ramana Maharshi[18]

Too much study of the scriptures does more harm than good. The important thing is to know the essence of the scriptures. After that, what is the need of books? One should learn the essence and then dive deep in order to realize God.

Sri Ramakrishna[19]

Svadhyaya means "self–study" and includes study of the sacred scriptures and teachings as well as the ego.

The studying of any teaching or philosophy is only productive for an individual to the degree that it can be applied in his or her daily life. As the readings' source often cautioned, knowledge not applied is sin (815–7, 254–93, 1456–1, for example). It is better not to know than to know and not act upon that knowledge. And so the readings state that with knowledge comes responsibility, because once you know, you are obligated to act in accordance with that knowledge.

In many cultures, one can find a heated diatribe between pundits and religious lawyers on the one hand and mystics on the other. The former worship the letter of the law, while the latter live the spirit of the law, which may not manifest in the way a pundit expects. The masters compel us to take *svadhyaya* into our own heart and allow intuition to mold and shape it. It is also helpful to get quality council from a wise teacher, one who has applied to self these same principles through repeated trial and error. Mere rhetoric is not the answer we seek.

Spiritual transformation—*inner* transformation—is the whole objective of a spiritual path, not what verses one has memorized or how many books one has read. Again, we can only transform ourselves to the degree that we apply the teachings in our daily lives, cultivating at the same time a greater awareness of how our ego is blocking our progress.

The readings' approach to *svadhyaya* is to study Scripture in order to "know thy relationship to the Creator." (1966–1) "Read [Scripture] not as history, . . . not as axioms or as dogmas, but as of thine own being." (1173–8)

If we look deeply enough into the ego, applying these timeless spiritual practices, we can discover the base unreality of the ego. It is a type of clever sensory illusion that has been ruling one's life. *Svadhyaya* is this process of distinguishing the ego from the Higher Self, or as it is commonly rendered in spiritual yoga, knowing the self from the Self.

V. Isvara-pranidhana

It is bad to stay in the church after you are grown up spiritually. Come out and die in the open air of freedom.   Swami Vivekananda

Blessed . . . is the man who is patient under trial and stands up under temptation, for when he has stood the test and been approved he will receive [the victor's] crown of life which God has promised to those who love Him.

James 1:12

So I have looked upon You in the sanctuary, to see Your power and Your glory. Because Your loving-kindness is better than life [itself] . . .   Psalm 63:2-3 [author's brackets]

God is love, and he who dwells and continues in love dwells and continues in God, and God dwells and continues in him.

1 John: 4:16

If a person [really] loves Me, he will keep my word [logos] . . . ; and My Father will love him, and We will come to him and make Our home . . . with him.

Jesus; John 14:23 [final brackets author's]

[As you] raise the consciousness to that within self, He [meets you] in [your] own tabernacle [of the body], in the holy of holies; in the third eye . . .   1782-1

In bhakti (devotional) yoga the central secret is . . . to know that the various passions and feelings and emotions in the human

heart are not wrong in themselves; they [just] have to be care-
fully controlled and given a higher and higher [spiritual] direction, until they attain the very highest condition of excellence.
The highest direction is that which takes us to God, every other
direction is lower.   Swami Vivekananda[20]

Therefore love God, not for His gifts, but because He is your
own, and because He made you in His image; and you will find
Him. If you meditate deeply, a love will come over you such as
no human tongue can describe; you will know His divine love,
and you will be able to give that love to others . . . True love is
divine, and divine love is joy. The more you meditate, seeking
God with a burning desire, the more you will feel that love in
your heart. Then you will know that love is joy, and joy is God.
                                              Paramahansa Yogananda[21]

Isvara-pranidhana is commonly translated as "surrender to God"; however, it would be more accurate to appreciate this concept as "surren-
der/devotion to the internal Lord." *Isvara* is the internal God, and to
pranam is to bow or supplicate oneself. This last component of the
niyamas reminds us that we cannot get too cerebral, or intellectual, about
the spiritual path—a critical part of spiritual awakening is to open one's
heart completely to Spirit, which is the ever-present substratum behind
one's individual consciousness. This *niyama* prompts us to fall in love
with Spirit, which can only realistically occur through consistent meditation and deconstruction of our many ego defenses.

The previous nine spiritual tenets are like the quality materials for a
fireplace and chimney. Without this last component, devotion (*Isvara-
pranidhana*), there is no fuel for the fire. It is devotion that ignites our
inner power and opens our awareness to higher realms. Once we commit to investing our heart, mind, and power in God consciousness, then
life takes on a new meaning and we start experiencing powerful awak-
enings.

The following excerpt from the readings incorporates many of the
yamas and *niyamas* in one piece of advice and is representative of the

particular way in which the readings' source implements spiritual yoga. So I return to this sentiment here, and again in a later chapter, because I think it is essential in understanding the bigger picture of spiritual development. Also, as a teaching contrivance, repetition (hopefully) breeds understanding, and it is important to understand that we are much more than mere eating and breathing machines.

> Man may not live by bread alone. Man may not live by the gratifying of appetites in the material world. For man is not made for this world alone. There is a longing for those experiences which the soul . . . has experienced. And without spirituality the earth is indeed a hell, an individual soul do what it will or may. Such longing may not be gratified from without or in the consciousness of . . . [external] forces and influences . . . For the body is indeed the temple of the living God. Act like it! Keep it clean. Don't desecrate it ever, but keep it such that it may be the place where you would meet [your] own better self, [your] own God-self. As [you] do this, there may be brought harmony, peace, joy. As in everything else, if [you] would have joy [you] must make others happy! Bring joy to others. If [you] would have love, [you] must show [yourself] lovely! If [you] would have friends, show yourself friendly! If [you] would know God, search for Him, for He is within [your] own self! And as [you] express Him in the fruits of spirit; love, grace, mercy, peace, longsuffering, patience, kindness, gentleness; [you] will find such within [yourself]. For if [you] would have life indeed (and life is the manifestation of God) [you] must give it. For the manner in which [you] treat [your] fellow man is the manner in which [you] treat [your] Maker. This is the source of life, the source of love, the source of peace, the source of harmony, and as [you] give expression to same, it may come indeed to [you].   4082-1

4

Meditation

Meditation is repeatedly emphasized in the Cayce readings and in the teachings of the Eastern masters. It is a skill that requires repetition and dedication to master. We are training our senses to withdraw while redirecting energy inward, to the source of consciousness, the source of life itself.

Meditation and the Readings

The readings' source frequently emphasizes meditation as the fundamental means to higher consciousness. The following excerpts in this section are taken from reading 281-13, one of the most comprehensive on the changes that occur during deep meditation.

> As has been given [in other readings], there are *definite* conditions that arise from within the inner man when an individual enters into true or deep meditation. A physical condition happens, a physical activity takes place! Acting through what? Through [what] man has chosen to call the imaginative or the impulsive, and the sources of impulse are aroused by the shutting out of thought pertaining to activities or attributes of the carnal forces of man. That is true whether we are considering it from the group standpoint or the individual.

Meditation changes you biochemically—it alters the functioning of hormones and neurotransmitters. In both group and individual meditation, the act of closing your eyes and redirecting thoughts has powerful spiritual benefits.

> Then, changes naturally take place when there is the arousing of [the] stimuli *within* the individual that has within it the seat of the soul's dwelling, within the individual body of the entity or man, and then this partakes of the individuality [soul level] rather than the personality [ego level].

Much of the time when people casually discuss "spiritual" activities, as in how they are involved or what they mean by the term, they actually are referring to philosophical activities on the ego level, not the spiritual. Understanding the spiritual in life requires awakening to the spirit, which is beyond the senses. Things that are spiritual pertain to an experience of one's soul-level existence, the subconscious and beyond, which transcends the sensory limitations.

> If there has been set the mark (mark meaning here the image that is raised by the individual in its imaginative and impulse force) such that it takes the form of the [spiritual] ideal the individual is holding as its standard to be raised to, within the individual as well as to all forces and powers that are magnified or to be magnified [externally] . . . *then* the individual (or the image) bears the mark of the Lamb, or the Christ, or the Holy One, or the Son, or any of the names we may have given to that which *enables* the individual to enter *through it* into the very presence of that which is the creative force from within itself—see?

Imagination is a very potent transformative power and grossly underestimated by many for its creative potential. Athletes and artists know that *if you can imagine it, you can create it*, and sages know that *if you believe it, you can achieve it*. This is because imagination *is* creation. The clearer your knowledge of what is pure and holy, the stronger you can magnetize your consciousness to become that. This is why the Cayce source states that your imagination will take hold of your spiritual ideal and create your reality, so it is essential to have a high spiritual ideal in order to really grow in consciousness.

> Some have so overshadowed themselves by abuses of the mental attributes of the body as to make scars, rather than the mark, so that only an imperfect image may be raised within themselves that may rise no higher than the arousing of the carnal desires within the individual body. We are speaking individually, of course; we haven't raised it to where it may be disseminated, for remember it rises from the glands known in the body as the lyden, or to the lyden [Leydig cells[22]] and through the reproductive forces themselves, which are the very essence of Life itself within an individual—see? for these functionings never reach that [condition] that they do not continue to secrete that which makes for virility to an individual physical body. Now we are speaking of conditions from without and from within!

Many people feed their mind garbage thoughts in the form of lust, greed, malice, fear, unworthiness, and arrogance, just to pick a few of the unsavory pieces off the top of the garbage pile. Because of this, they cannot raise spiritual energies to the higher centers. That is why the *yamas* and *niyamas* are so crucial to higher consciousness—they purify the mind for deeper states of spiritual attunement. The more the *yamas* and *niyamas* are faithfully lived, the greater the propensity to raise spiritual vibrations.

> The spirit and the soul is within its encasement, or its temple within the body of the individual—see? With the arousing then of this image [the spiritual ideal], it rises along that which is known as the Appian Way [the spinal cord], or the pineal center, to the base of the *brain*, that it may be disseminated to those centers [chakras] that give activity to the whole of the mental and physi-

cal being. It rises then to the hidden eye in the center of the
brain system, or is felt in the forefront of the head [the "third
eye"], or in the place just above the real face—or bridge of
nose, see?

The spine has a central canal called the *sushumna* through which
spiritual energies rise from the sacrum (tailbone) to the brain. As the
energies make their upward ascent, they activate each spiritual center,
or *chakra*, along the way. The end of upward flow is at the junction of
three important "mini–factories" in the brain: the pineal, hypothalamus,
and pituitary gland. These three small structures basically control the
whole functionality of the body. When we focus on the Christ center,
located between the eyes (the "third eye"), we are using willpower to
magnetize the spine and raise the spinal energies to the highest chakras.
This is the literal meaning of *raising one's consciousness*.

When an individual then enters into deep meditation:

It has been found throughout the ages (*individuals* have found)
that self-preparation (to *them*) is necessary. To some it is necessary that the body be cleansed with pure water, that certain
types of breathing are taken, that there may be an even balance
in the whole of the respiratory system, that the circulation becomes normal in its flow through the body, that certain or defi-
nite odors produce those conditions (or are conducive to
producing of conditions) that allay or stimulate the activity of
portions of the system, that the more carnal or more material
sources are laid aside, or the whole of the body is *purified* so
that the purity of thought as it rises has less to work against in
its dissemination of [energies] it brings to the whole of the system, in its rising through the whole of these centers, stations or
places along the body. To be sure, these are conducive; as are
also certain incantations, as a drone of certain sounds, as the
tolling of certain tones, bells, cymbals, drums . . . Though we
may [from a spiritual vantage] find some fault with those called

> savages, [who] produce or arouse . . . within . . . the battle-cry,
> there may be raised through the using of certain words or [de-
> vices], the passion or the thirst for destructive forces. [In] just
> the same [way] may there be raised, not sedative [energies] but
> a *cleansing* of the body.

The readings insist on a ritual "cleansing" before entering meditation.
This is a preparatory phase that can take many forms: bathing,
breathwork, and chanting are the most commonly employed throughout various traditions. The last part of this section explains that in the
same way "savages" can work themselves into a destructive frenzy for
conflict by ruminating on a thought, the spiritual aspirant can use this
same intensity as a means to purify the mind. Both music and chanting
install messages into one's subconscious—so be very discriminating as
to what you put there.

> When one has found that which . . . cleanses the body, whether
> from the keeping away from certain foods or from certain
> [sexual] associations (either man or woman), or from those
> thoughts and activities that would hinder [the spiritual energies]
> . . . to be raised, . . . we readily see how, then, *in* meditation
> (when one has so purified self) that *healing of every* kind and
> nature may be disseminated on the wings of thought, [which is
> very real] . . . and so little considered by the tongue that speaks
> without taking into consideration what may be the end thereof!

It is when one's consciousness is purified that healing can occur. Just
remember that healing, according to the readings, is the result of attuning self to God consciousness; you don't meditate just for a physical
healing but to be closer in consciousness to Spirit.

> Now, when one has cleansed self, in whatever manner it may
> be, there may be no fear that it will become so overpowering
> that it will cause any physical or mental disorder. It is *without*
> the cleansing that [a person] entering [into a deep meditative

state may find] *any* type or form of disaster, or of pain, or of any dis-ease of any nature. It is when [one's] thoughts, then, or when the cleansings of *group* meditations are conflicting that such meditations call on the higher forces raised within self for [physical] manifestations and bring those conditions that either draw one closer to another or make for that which shadows . . . much in the experiences of others; hence short group meditations with a *central* thought around some individual idea, or either in words, incantations, or by following the speech of one sincere in abilities, efforts or desires to raise a cooperative activity *in* the minds, would be the better.

Because our minds can veer off during meditation (and certainly will in the beginning stages), it is important to practice a method of meditation that teaches how to focus. Learning how to concentrate your mind in one spot and keep it there for an extended period of time is the basis of *samyama*, the final stages of enlightenment yoga. When engaged in group meditation, it is effective to have the group focus on a common affirmation, chant, or prayer. This becomes the group's focus and makes it easier for each individual to hold to that common thought.

Cleanse the body with pure water. Sit or lie in an easy position, without binding garments about the body. Breathe in through the right nostril three times, and exhale through the mouth. Breathe in three times through the left nostril and exhale through the right. Then, either with the aid of a low music, or the incantation of that which carries self deeper—deeper—to the seeing, feeling, experiencing of that image in the creative forces of love, enter into the Holy of Holies. As self feels or experiences the raising of this, see it disseminated through the *inner* eye (not the carnal eye) to that which will bring the greater understanding in meeting every condition in the experience of the body. Then listen to the music that is made as each center of [your] own body responds to that new creative force that little by little . . . will enable self to renew all that is necessary—in Him.

It is imperative that the meditator's clothes not restrict circulation; if blood is not flowing well, then neither is vital energy. The breathing exercise recommended balances the left and right currents of the spine and the two cerebral hemispheres, respectively. The "Holy of Holies" is the Christ center, in between the eyes. Your eyes naturally go to that point every night in sleep. The changes that occur in the body happen little by little, which is why repetition and regularity of practice are important.

> Prayer is the concerted effort of the physical consciousness to become attuned to the consciousness of the Creator, either collectively or individually! *Meditation* is *emptying* self of all that hinders the creative forces from rising along the natural channels of the physical man to be disseminated through those centers and sources that create the activities of the physical, the mental, the spiritual man; properly done must make one *stronger* mentally, physically, for has it not been given? He went in the strength of that meat received for many days? Was it not given by Him who has shown us the Way, "I have had meat that ye know not of"? As we give out, so does the *whole* of man— physically and mentally become depleted, yet in entering into the silence, entering into the silence in meditation, with a clean hand, a clean body, a clean mind, we may receive that strength and power that fits each individual, each soul, for a greater activity in this material world.   281-13

Prayer directs willpower to spiritual realms, while meditation is receiving both the increase in vital energy up the spine and the "strength and power" of higher consciousness. Many great yogis have demonstrated remarkable power over physical phenomena by using mental and energetic techniques. They have also demonstrated that food is not our only source of energy. As a matter of fact, both Jesus and the mahayogis state that vital energy is our real food.

There are various energetic phenomena that occur in meditation. These should not be overly emphasized or forced to occur. Movements of the body are natural byproducts of the sacred spinal energies rising.

One phenomenon, sometimes called "angel's kisses," occurs with the feeling of coolness upon the forehead. A woman in the readings who experienced this "breath of an angel" was told that through attunement, she would

> be a channel where there may be even instant healing with the laying on of hands. The more often this occurs the more power is there felt in the body, the forcefulness in the act or word.
>
> 281-5

A common phenomenon is for the body to move, rocking back and forth or in a circular manner, while the mind is internally focused. The readings' source recommends being aware of whether this is self-created or not. If it is self-generated, if a person is willing this to happen, it is suggested that it be controlled in order to deepen the attunement. If it is not self-generated—if it is occurring through no voluntary control of the meditator—then the recommendation is to surrender to it and deepen one's

Yoga is impossible unless the mind becomes quiet.   Sri Ramakrishna

attunement (that is, don't focus on the external, but increase the internal attunement).

Meditation is Attuning One's Consciousness to God's Frequency

[W]ith each material manifestation [incarnation] there is an undertaking by an entity to so manifest as [to] become more and more attuned to that consciousness [of God].   2533-1

There He—as all knowledge, all undertakings, all wisdom, all understanding—may commune with thee . . . By attuning, turning thy thought, thy purpose, thy desire to be at an at-onement with Him.   2533-4

As is seen in all of the forms of vibration, whether in the mineral, in the vegetable, in the animal, in music, in . . . chemicals, or those of spiritual vibrations . . . [I]f the body is made animal by the excess . . . gratification of animal desires, [the vibrations] become of the lower vibration. If [that attunement] is made . . . with the bodies celestial, bodies terrestrial, or of whatever form—these develop through that same vibration . . . To that vibration [to which] one attunes self, that [same] response [returns].   256-2

Keep the face toward the *light*, keeping self in attune to that Oneness wherein all power, and all force, is at the command of the entity in applying those forces known within self to meet the needs of each and every condition.   39-4

There is no cure-all [for diseases] except being in attune[ment] with the Infinite.   658-15

Chanting

[I]n all of thy meditation, Ohm—o-h-m-m-mmmmm has ever been, is ever a portion of that which raises self to the highest influence and the highest vibrations throughout its whole being that may be experienced . . .   1286-1

. . . following that known in thine own present as i-e-o-u-e-i-o-umh . . . for the raising of that from within of the Creative Forces, as it arises along that . . . cord of life . . . , that balance between the mind, the body, the soul . . .   275-43

In the Gnostic tract *The Gospel of the Egyptians*, there is a passage that closely resembles Cayce's chanting recommendation:

The Father of the great light who came forth from the silence, he is the great Doxomedon-aeon in which the thrice-male child rests. And the throne of his glory was established in it, this one on which his unrevealable name is inscribed on the tablet . . . one is the word, the Father of the light of everything, he who came forth from the silence, while he rests in the silence, he whose name is in an invisible symbol. A hidden, invisible mystery came forth: iiiiiiiiiii, eeeeeeeeeeee, ooooooooooooo, uuuuuuuuu, eeeeeeee, aaaaaaaaa, ooooooooooooooooooo.[23]

Meditation in the Yogic Traditions

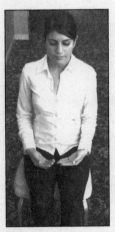

Meditation is the cornerstone of spiritual yoga. The entire point of all the yogic practices is to transcend self, to rise above the facades of the ego.

The correct posture is to sit with the back straight but not tense, away from the chair's backrest. (See photos 1 and 2.) The pressure against the back of the body can prevent the subtle spinal energies from moving efficiently. (See photos 3 and 4.) Keep your chest in the neutral position, not concave (see photo 4), which will align your skull over your collarbones. You want the spine straight, from the tailbone to the back of the skull, so do not slouch forward. Place your forearms on your thighs, palms upward. This is a position of receptivity and makes a difference in the quality of your meditation. (See photo 2.) Once this posture is established and you know you are sitting with a straight and relaxed spine, head directly over the shoulders, forget about the body and completely focus on the breath.

In breathing, you should slowly inhale through the nose and breathe out through the mouth with a relaxed jaw, expanding your lower abdomen and not your upper chest. With eyes closed, synchronize your inhalation with the thought "Be still." You are not saying this but *thinking* it for the full length of the inhalation. Next, synchronize your exhalation with the thought "Know God." This first stage of meditation is for deepening this breath-thought synchronization to a point that you lose track of time, space, and the body.

Next, focus your gaze on the point between the eyes, slightly higher than your eyebrow line. This is the Christ Consciousness center. Continue the breath-thought synchronization while allowing for more space between inhalation and exhalation. Slow down all processes. Absorb yourself in the natural energy found at this point. Eventually, a sense of light and joy emerge, and this signifies that you are attuning deeper. There is a joyful light here that starts as a tiny bead and eventually expands—all in relation to the purity of your consciousness and the intensity of your introspection.

Correct position

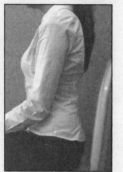 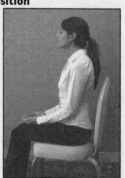

Photograph 1   Photograph 2

Incorrect position

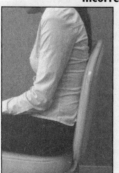 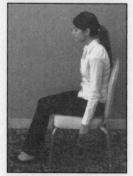

Photograph 3   Photograph 4

Photos by Istvan Fazekas.
Model: Stephanie Rountree.

5

12 *Steps to Enlightenment*
According to the Cayce Readings

Step 1: Harmony

Let the body learn that, he that would have harmony must be harmonious first within his own self, and such radiation from self will bring to the home, to business, to friends, such a peace that brings harmonious contentment – [and though you may not be fully] *satisfied* . . . be *content* with that *in* hand, and so act, so live, and so manifest harmony through self's action as to bring [inner and outer harmony] to pass; for what is sown one also reaps. When the act—either by physical deed, implication or word—is such as to put even the question mark as to what is the intent and purpose, dissatisfaction is created; and remember, thoughts are *deeds* and may become crimes or miracles! Apply that in the relations [within] the home, and the harmony . . .

sought will be the outcome. Not with an eye-service of, "that I
may have my own way", or "that I may bring others to *my* own
way of acting, or own way of thinking"; but let [your] thought,
[your] act, be so in harmony with that of the inner life as to
radiate harmony; for when one looks about in all nature . . . the
first law is harmony, and is of divine origin, even as life, and
when [one] is not in accord *with* . . . the Creative Energy, or God,
discord is the result.   4733-1

The idea of the "first law" appears in the readings in a few contexts.
Although it may initially appear that the readings' source is presenting
various "first laws," I think it is instead presenting different layers of one
philosophical continuum—the idea that all things are connected. This
helps us further define and understand the concept of harmony. The
individual must be in harmony with the tribe, tribes must be in harmony with other tribes, and mankind must live in harmony with nature.

The idea of self-protection is presented as a first law in reading 759-
13 and others. In this context, it means that among many earthly "laws,"
or biological and physiological necessities—survival, procreation, personal safety, tribal security, and so on—self-protection comes as a primary concern. But expanding out from there, we can see that since we
are all connected, essentially different expressions of one animating
Spirit, to injure another is simply self-punishment. This moves us to the
readings' bigger philosophical lesson that *like attracts like* and that everything is one (connected in God's matrix).

This is looking at the big picture from the microcosm (personal survival) out toward the macrocosm. But, if we invert the lens, starting
with the macrocosm, we get this message from reading 1527-3, "The
Lord thy God is One!" Everything that is occurring amongst the complex interactions of various life forms, and of mind shaping physical
reality, is the result of the complicated interplay of God's will. And,
although there is one Force behind all this, it is so enormous and has so
many facets to its matrix that it is often easier to relate to it in pieces—
angels, laws of gravity and electromagnetism, various spiritual strata,

astronomical movements, cellular biology, and so forth. The readings remind us time and again that, although Creative Forces operate through multiple manifestations, there is one phenomenon occurring within and around us—God.

In order for us to be in harmony with God, we must be in harmony as an individualized unit of God; we must have body, mind, and spirit all working together on a continuous basis. This is where we start in understanding Cayce's law of harmony.

The first law of the sages and the readings' source is to live and act with a purpose of creating harmony within and without. This is the intention of the sacred *yamas* and *niyamas*. We are put on earth to be catalysts for goodness, helpfulness, service, and enlightenment to others. We do not have to be perfect but ever ready to lend a hand to a person in need—whether it be material, psychological, or spiritual assistance another seeks. In all our imperfection and faltering, we can still be, and should be, of service to others.

Harmony is the first law, because we are all individual cells in the body of God. If one cell goes awry, then others may follow, leading to a symbolic tumor in society. We have many levels of bodies here: the global body, the continental body, the national body, the provincial body, the familial body, and the individual body. They are all connected in various ways. The sages have taught for centuries that if enough people committed themselves to individual peace and spiritual attunement, it would have a radiating influence on the other bodies, eventually leading to healing the global body. So in a very real and tangible way, world peace starts with inner peace—global harmony starts with individual harmony.

The opening reading (4733-1) to this chapter addresses harmony on its most pragmatic level. For many people, their version of *harmonious* means to make others conform to their way of being or thinking. This is not spiritualized harmony. True harmony means to know intuitively what is best for all parties concerned and to understand how to minimize the ego in order to allow Spirit to work through one's consciousness. What the Cayce source labels as "eye-service," we could modify to "I-service." It is our I-service that constantly rearranges a given situation to adapt it to our personal needs, instead of meeting the situation on its own terms and allowing Spirit to resolve factors, aligning them with the big picture.

All harmony must first begin as an inner discovery and end as a social act:

> *The more one regards the feelings of others, the more harmony one can create.   Hazrat Inayat Khan*

> Then, the first law of knowing self, of understanding self, is to become more and more sincere with that thou doest in the relationships one to another. For the proof of same is the fruit thereof.
> 261-15

> *It is not a particular religion that can produce spirituality in man; spirituality depends upon the tuning of the soul.   Hazrat Inayat Khan*

We are asked to develop a better sense of our usefulness to the community in which we live. How sincere are we one to another? Having a mind-set to simply sell something to others without considering their needs or interests is not sincerity but tantamount to proselytizing.

The law of cause and effect applies to each situation in which we seek harmony: If we want understanding, we must first understand; if we want forgiveness, we must first forgive; if we want prosperity for ourselves, we must first be a source of prosperity for others; if we want Spirit to guide us, we must first be guidable by learning to be silent and meditative.

As we have seen with the *yama* of *ahimsa*, active nonviolence is a divine law of the Universe—it is the way the Creative Forces operate. God does not use force to change you but instead employs the impartial law of karma, under which everyone is equally subject. We, too, are asked to keep this in mind in our dealings with one another.

> For it is a unison of desire that brings a seeking at any time for expression, and *not* in *combative* reactions at all! For when there is the combative self-assertion, egotism and selfishness rise to

the forefront *as* that ordinarily known as self-protection—which
is a first law [or primitive response].

But as long as there is kept that unison, correct—as long as
there is that *great* activity which all should know. If the world will
ever know its best, it must learn *cooperation!* . . .

Yet if there is the attempt—as has been indicated—to have
self's way (the egotism, the self-expression), [you] defeat the
First Law [that we are all one].   759-13

Some people are under the misunderstanding that they could not
possibly function in this world if their ego were minimized. This is like
a baby chick thinking that it could not possibly function in this world
without its hard, protective eggshell. Perhaps a certain chick is under
the delusion that the shell is itself and that by cracking the shell, it too
will crack. Until it becomes brave enough to break out of that shell,
which served a purpose for a predetermined time, it will always stay
inside and never live to be what it was created for. We're the same.

We are perfect spirits trapped
inside the delusion of the ego.
The "shell," in our case, is the
mind—the habits and attachments we create with our free
will. One manifestation of the
ego—fear—is a powerful force
that keeps people living on a
lower energetic plane. The fear of
pain is often worse than the pain
itself, especially since our bodies

> The secret of seeking the will of
> God lies in cultivating the faculty of
> sensing harmony; for harmony is
> beauty and beauty is harmony . . .
> and by trying always to maintain
> harmony, man will tune his heart to
> the will of God.
>
> *Hazrat Inayat Khan*

are equipped with intrinsic neurochemicals thousands of times more
potent than heroin. The fear of loss is worse than the loss itself; many
terrible acts have been committed by humans trying to avoid loss. The
fear of dying motivates many to commit useless acts meant to save
them from the inevitable, when the truth is that death is a natural and
beautiful transition. Ask anyone who has had a near–death experience,
and such an experiencer will tell you that dying was easy and that the

newfound, out-of-body state of consciousness was exceptionally satisfying. It is being here on earth that is filled with challenges, but these
challenges are immensely valuable to our soul growth and should not
be discounted or belittled; it is a very precious opportunity to be on
earth and to learn and to grow. Understanding harmony means to keep
awareness that we are all here on earth for the central purpose of learning and growing. We are asked to take care of one another in the process.

Spiritual maturity allows one to reframe life's challenges and see them
as opportunities to practice the spiritual disciplines and occasions to
surrender to Spirit. Only the spiritually immature run from responsi-
bilities. Eventually, the realization occurs that there is nowhere to run,
as the cat cannot get away from its own tail no matter how fast it sprints.
Everywhere you go, there you are—so where are you going?

> As we may find in a material world: Envy, strife, selfishness,
> greediness, avarice, are the children of *man!* Longsuffering,
> kindness, brotherly love, good deeds, are the children of the
> spirit of light.   5753-1

> [H]e that may not cooperate one with another has little part in
> that that may be accomplished; for whether these be much or
> little, *their* activity—in *accord*—keeps harmony; harmony
> makes for peace; peace for understanding; understanding for
> enlightenment. In *this*, then, let *all* be active.   262-4

6

12 Steps to Enlightenment According to the Cayce Readings

Step 2: Consistent Meditation

Be still and know that I am God . . .   Psalm 46:10 [KJV]

Have God first. Have God now. Don't wait, because delusion is very strong. Before you know it, the time will have come for you to quit this world. Whenever you have a moment, sit down and meditate.   Paramahansa Yogananda[24]

Attain [the] highest consciousness by deep meditation, and this highest consciousness will be [your] perfect master.

Baba Hari Dass

Because the subject of meditation is the only topic repeated in the *A Search for God* books, developed by Mr. Cayce and his associates, it is repeated here but with additional information. Most people are highly uninformed about the importance of meditation to their enlightenment. Consistently meditating is, without a doubt, one of the most important activities to bring you into a greater awareness of Spirit—it is the basis for authentic spirituality.

The difference between prayer and meditation is explained numerous ways in the readings. The distinction is important in order to maximize the effectiveness of each.

Prayer is

- Setting a sincere spiritual intention
- Humbling the ego by surrendering to Spirit
- Giving thanks for being a channel of blessing, for being guided by Creative Forces, and for life challenges that are working out one's karma
- Expressing joy and gratitude for Spirit's wonderfully mysterious and mysteriously wonderful activities
- Cleansing the heart and mind as a preparation for meditation
- The directing of spiritual intention, after meditation, for others' healing or enlightenment

Meditation is

- Listening deeply to God's activity and stillness within
- Clearing one's mind of obstructive static
- Attuning the body–mind to God
- Raising one's vibrations: the process of *kundalini shakti,* arising in the spine
- Time to allow God to love and recharge you
- Perfect stillness of body and mind, which eventually facilitates an indescribable bliss—an indication of proximity to higher consciousness

Benefits of meditation

- Calms and balances the nervous system
- Positively affects the endocrine system
- Increases the vividness and recall of dreams
- Helps one get into deeper sleep states faster, helping remedy insomnia
- Finely tunes one's intuition
- Gives actual experience of God consciousness as a joyful, peaceful presence of Light and spaciousness
- Helps one see through one's mental machinations
- With repeated practice, eventually exposes the unreality of the ego

The readings' approach to meditation is related to the yogic *bhakti* path—unconditional surrender to God and cultivation of transpersonal love. For many Hindus, the object of their devotion would be Krishna; for Cayce, the choice is the Christ. Both are icons of the Higher Self.

> For, know—as He hath given – "Lo, I am with thee always, even unto the end." This is not a mere saying, but an awareness which one may find through that attuning through meditation, through prayer, through the opening of self for direction by Him.
>
> 69-4

Cultivating the habit of daily meditation, for numerous aspirants, is the most difficult discipline. At first, it is a labor, but after reaping the many benefits of meditation, it becomes something one looks forward to—it is a delightful and necessary oasis in the desert of life.

There are many activities that may enrich our minds and character, but the regular practice of meditation facilitates the greatest spiritual development: "[Meditate] Once a day, at least." (257-149)

Meditation must be made a habit by repetition. The readings' recommendation is to choose a time of day or night for regular meditation

and stay to that. If you set a time
to meditate, it is more likely that
you will make it a habit. If you
say, "I'll get to it sometime later,"
odds are that that time will be
filled with something else. In an-

> *We are always searching for God far
> off, when all the while He is nearer
> to us than our soul.*
>
> *Hazrat Inayat Khan*

cient traditions and in the readings, just before dawn and right after
dusk are two energetically powerful times to meditate, but if these times
are not practical for you, choose a time that is.

There is a chain reaction that occurs with meditation—gaining inner
peace brings you closer to others, which leads to understanding, which
leads to higher vibrational living.

> In the meditations—we would set as a specific time for all to
> meditate; for he that may not cooperate one with another has
> little part in that that may be accomplished; for whether these
> be much or little, *their* activity—in *accord*—keeps harmony;
> harmony makes for peace; peace for understanding; under-
> standing for enlightenment. In *this*, then, let *all* be active.
>
> 262-4

Eventually, one's meditation time is not so removed from daily life.
The internal spiritual focus gets brought into everyday awareness:

> [W]e become more conscious of His presence abiding with us,
> as we let that mind—through meditation and prayer—be in us
> during and at *all* periods.   262-33

We cannot be guided by Spirit if we have the pesky ego–mind inter-
fering. Meditation makes our intuitive awareness more acute, which
lifts our consciousness closer to God.

> Hence, set a portion [of time for the] communing with the inner
> [S]elf through meditation and prayer to the Giver of all good and
> perfect gifts; knowing there is a mediator that ever stands ready

to make intercession, and He has given those promises that anywhere, any time that the soul calls, He *will* harken, He will guide. 274-3

Be oft, then, in prayer, in meditation, in love, in communion of body, of mind, of soul, that the Father may have His way with thee. 294-174

One improper approach to meditation is trying to force some kind of vision or sign. This is *not* the point of meditation; it is highly erroneous and should be discarded in favor of simply surrendering to Spirit. The other problem for many is that they read too much about meditation or listen to others' experiences, and this prejudices them against what is naturally there within. Do not expect others' experiences to be replicated by you—find your own experiences by going within. The essential point of meditation is to just *be*—cultivating stillness, peace, and inner awareness—being present with whatever you find.

> *Until the heart is empty, it cannot receive the knowledge of God.*
> Hazrat Inayat Khan

In this reading, the Cayce source explains why a woman is having problems meditating:

Oft we find individual activity becomes so personal in even the meditations that there is sought that this or that, which may have been reported to have happened to another, *must* be the manner of happening to self. And in this manner there is cut away, there is built the barrier which prevents the real inner self from *experiencing*. Let self *loose*, as it were; for [your] prayer ascends to the throne of grace, ever; only as self, though, [gives] out to [your] fellow man. Do not *try*, or crave, or desire a sign; for [you are] in *[your]self* a sign of that [which you] worship within [your] inner self! For [you], as every soul, [do] stand before the door of the temple where [your] God [has] promised to

meet [you]. Then, do not be impatient. For what [you ask] in
secret shall be proclaimed from the housetop.   705-2

As will become apparent, one cannot expect meditation alone to
eradicate poor behavior. The authentic spiritual path is a marriage between ethics/morals, service, surrender, and introspection/self-tran-
scendence. We could also say this is the foundation for all true religion.

Keep the body, the mind, the whole of the intent and purpose
circumspect; not as to what others say but as to what your
conscience—in prayer, in meditation—may show you. For as
He has given, "My Spirit beareth witness with thy spirit." This is
the answer then to each soul.   1089-7

Physical changes occur as the result of regular meditation. One
should not get focused on the physical phenomena, imaginative activities, or even wanting to see visions. The more centered you remain
during meditation, the more you can work through all the many layers
of ego consciousness, which is where any notion of your becoming
"enlightened" or being "spiritual" is originating. Remember: You do not
need to add something to yourself to find the Light . . . you need to
systematically discard all the unenlightened parts.

The ego is going to play many tricks on you until you gain inner
strength. The first step is to focus on just one holy thought and absorb
your consciousness into it. If the ego habits veer your mind off into
chimerical fantasies, shopping lists, interpersonal dramas, and so forth,
then you must bring it back a thousand times or a thousand times a
thousand until you eventually see beyond this.

Meditation reveals the essence of mysticism, the meeting point of all
holy traditions. The following
reading mentions both Socrates
and the Buddha as meditators.   *The deeper your prayers echo in*
The legacy of both of these spiri-   *your own consciousness, the more*
tual giants is still being felt to-   *audible they are to God.*
day. Both were mystics and both   *Hazrat Inayat Khan*

contacted the Source through meditation:

> Socrates, as he meditated . . . And . . . [the] Buddha, in that
> position when meditation in the forest brought to the conscious-
> ness of the entity the At-Oneness of *all force* manifested through
> physical aspects, or physical, in a material world.   900-187

As the sages assert, there is an element of grace involved in higher
states of realization. All the effort falls on your shoulders, as you are
given will to use wisely, but Spirit's grace is necessary for advanced
stages of spiritual transformation. One's grace expands, or compounds,
as spiritual activity builds on itself.

> For we grow in grace, in knowledge, in understanding *from
> within*. And even though there are the words of the mouth, even
> the activities of the body, if they are done, if they are *meditated*
> upon to be seen [by others], to be feeling, to be making only an
> outward show, these must eventually come to [nothing]. For the
> *kingdom* is within. Contentment, peace, harmony, glory, love,
> beauty, [comes] from *within*; and is as a growth [development]
> that makes for that activity, that expression, that which will bring
> the growth, the understanding, the environments, the neces-
> sary influences [we require to develop God consciousness]. For
> with all the labors, the efforts, with all the application of beauty,
> of strength, of power, of might, *only* God may give the increase.
> 165-21

All meetings with Spirit start as a connection between the conscious
and subconscious. It requires introspection and the shutting out of sensory habits that obscure the subtleties of God. The following excerpts
on meditation are taken from reading 261-15.

> Then, in making practical or concrete [spiritual activities in your]
> experience, first enter in . . . through the meditative forces within
> self; through the purifying of the body, of the mind, that it may

be one and in accord, in attune[ment] with the Creative Forces from within; setting the ideal in Him who has promised to meet [you] in the holy of holies, in the temple of [your] soul, in [your] own body-consciousness.

> *We seek religion because we want to do away with our suffering forever. Worldly methods are not the answer. God is the answer; true religion that brings God-realization is the answer. So now is the time to wake up; take the sword of wisdom and slash away all bad habits.*
>
> *Yogananda*

Once again, the emphasis is placed upon the quality of our actions—practicing the *yamas* and *niyamas* in daily life. Our actions and our worship are two wheels on the same chariot of consciousness. Anyone who thinks one can be pious and devoted on a Sunday and then a social bane on Monday, without expecting repercussions, is only fooling oneself:

Thus does the self, the I AM, become aware of that presence. And in meeting day by day in the walks with [your] fellow man, sow those seeds that *[you]* would reap in [your] experience. For they, the seeds [which you] sow, [you] *become*—as it were . . . ! For each soul meets that [which] it has [doled out or inflicted upon] the fellow man. For as He gave, "As ye do it unto the least of these, my little ones, ye do it unto me."

There is a subtle magnetism that occurs in deep meditation: you are both sending and receiving this energy once you can control your mental waves. As previously mentioned, the external manifestations of Spirit occur as the result of internal transformations:

Psychic is of the soul, then, first becoming aware of its inactivity or activity toward the Creator within [your] own experience. Not as from without; for the external experiences will be the natural result when the self is attuned [to Spirit]. As [you] attune [your] own mechanical instruments to the vibrations of this or that sending influence, [you] receive that which is being sent out or vibrated *upon* that plane.

[Such is the same with your] body . . . mind . . . soul, as the sending, as the receiving, as the giving forth in [your] activities and [your] walks before men.

Practicing the *yamas* and *niyamas* sanctifies your body–mind, preparing you for spiritual experiences. When you vibrate at a lower modulation, living selfishly in the first three chakras, you can only experience things that relate to that level of awareness. In order for higher awareness to occur, we must change our inner view, and the outer view follows:

This, then, is the manner. Enter . . . in at the gate called straight, through [your] own preparation in [your] own manner, and meet Him there [within]. For [your] body is the temple of the living God, of [your] living soul; [your] body is the temple that must be, should be, *will* be kept holy, if [you] will know [your] true relationships to [your] Maker.   261-15

The fewer expectations you have in meditation the better, as expectations activate the mind, sending you down the road to ten thousand thoughts. Focus on perfect stillness and allow self-transcendence to naturally develop. Let your personal agendas dissolve, and immerse yourself completely in that Inner Light, found at the Christ center, between the eyes. Put the burden of your life completely on God's shoulders, and relish in that time of fervent surrender. The readings recommend that you mentally surround yourself in a white light and hold to the Christ Ideal as a kind of energetic cleansing, or protection, prior to meditating.

Most people impetuously seek happiness in external things. They seek and never find. The happiness they think they have found in that property, gadget, cuisine, or person soon fades. Too few know that the happiness they *really* want is found only by diving deeply within their own consciousness to the core of their existence. There will be layers of neuroses, or mental waves, to have to work through, but the effort is well worth the eventual reward of inner clarity and inner peace. No one else can do this inner work for you, and no external person, place, or thing will suffice.

Once you have reached the point of calming the mental storm that plagues so many, you can move to the next level: entering into the heart. The mind can only take you so far, but the heart can take you into the deepest realms of true spirituality. The heart is a powerful engine, with wings that open to the Infinite. Focus on the heart in meditation—soften and deepen that place. You can experience it as a portal through which the greatest beauty and ecstasy can be felt. But even here, at this sublime and wonderful stage, we must move deeper, past the impossible joy, and enter into a land of perfect stillness and spaciousness. This is the way of the masters, and the ideal journey.

7

12 *Steps to Enlightenment*
According to the Cayce Readings

Step 3: Self-Study

The recommendation to "know thyself" arises numerous times in the Cayce readings. A common maxim that occurs in one form or another is, "Know *yourself* to *be* yourself and yet one with God." (281-37) Many people have very limiting or misleading self-identifications—they do not know

What is ever the worst fault of each soul? *Self—self!* . . .

For the only sin of man is *selfishness* . . . [This may be overcome by] showing mercy . . . grace . . . peace, longsuffering, brotherly love, kindness—even under the most *trying* circumstances.   987-4

that there is a spirit inhabiting a "costume" with a particular (and temporary) gender, nationality, race, religious creed, and so on. Many erroneously think they *are* their costume.

Self-study is the primary interpretation of *svadhyaya*. The readings recommend self-study coupled with Bible study. In the yogic tradition, studying the sacred texts also has a place. As the masters counsel, one should devote more time to internally reflecting on religious/spiritual rhetoric and prose than to reading passages. Self-study brings wisdom and genuine understanding to the ideas found in the sacred texts.

In a reading for developing the Search for God material, the readings' source states, "The kingdom, then, is within. Go. Do." (262-12) This is very much in line with Asian spiritual traditions that emphasize action over mere rhetoric.

Self-study includes examining yourself as others see you. In some clinical therapies, when the objective is behavior modification, people are video/audiotaped in the midst of their unhealthy behavior. Most often the subjects are shocked to see just how careless, cruel, malicious, or tactless they come across to others. Some even insist that it must be someone else, not themselves. This is because, while deeply immersed in ego consciousness, we are like a sleepwalker, deeply unaware of the Presence behind our consciousness. How can we aspire to understand God when we don't even know ourselves?

One analogy used in the yogic traditions to help explain this is the fisherman standing in the muddy river. If a fisherman is trying to locate fish to catch, he needs to find the placid waters where the fish can be clearly observed from above the waterline. If he starts to run about, kicking up sediment underwater, he will cloud the water and scare away the fish. This is what we do by remaining in ego consciousness—we keep muddying the waters and scaring away the fish of peacefulness and spiritual lucidity. Meditation and self-study help calm the restless mental waves that perpetuate our unmindful behavior and ego immersion.

In this reading for a twenty-one-year-old female student, the counsel given covers a few yogic principles:

[Y]et for the greater development keep first the understanding of self and self's relationship to others first and foremost [practice correct svadhyaya]. Beware of entanglements with those of

the opposite sex [practice rightful brahmacharya] . . . Beware
of conditions as pertaining to bodily ills that have to do with the
digestive system [live dietary shauca]. Keep self unspotted from
low relationships, and keep thyself bodily clean [employ interpersonal and somatic shauca].   169-1

Another common piece of advice in the readings is shown in the
following reading, presenting the readings' version of *svadhyaya* and
encouraging the forty–two–year–old Jewish secretary to show herself
"approved unto God, a workman not ashamed":

First, study to show thyself approved unto God, a workman not
ashamed, rightly divining—or dividing—the words of truth; that
is, giving proper evaluations to the material, the mental and the
spiritual relationships, the economic, the social, the orders of
things in their proper form.
   Be not hasty in decisions but know that the answers may
come from within . . .
   Keep self unspotted from the world of thine own consciousness, condemning none—and most of all not self. God loveth
the cheerful giver.   189-3

The next excerpt is another example of how the readings' source can
be at par with yogic counsel:

This should be the attitude of self: Make self *selfless*. He that
will humble himself will be exalted. Do not run away from the
shadows of self. When self takes counsel, or when self goes
aside and takes stock of the conditions and experiences that
have been in the life of self, have not most of them been caused
by that fear, or that condemnation that has been held in the
inner man respecting the manner in which self has been treated
at home? Has not that abroad been the same? With what measure ye mete, with what condemnation ye make, so shall it be
measured to you again! [You] cannot *hide* [yourself] in numbers

[crowds], in running away to distant places or anywhere! *Self* is ever in the presence of the godly conditions of [your] making. If [your] ideal is set in the material things, only material things can be the reaping or the harvest. If [your] ideal is set in higher things, and [your] acts day by day are in [alignment with your ideal], then the harvest may be expected to be in that proportion commensurate with that given. Measure self not by self, for who[ever] does [so] is unwise. [Don't condemn yourself or others] . . . Know in *whom* there is hope, for it comes only from the answering of a pure conscience from within. Ask not who will ascend to bring peace and harmony from on high, or where shall I go to seek peace and harmony abroad? *Know it must be created within [your] own heart, and soul!* [Your] own self must answer to [your] Maker with an all-good conscience. When self can look the world and all straight in the face, and move on towards the better things, forgetting that which is [in the past], moving on to the higher forces that [create true] faith, confidence, and of the purposes that will be set before thee from day to day, then the inner [self] will find peace, harmony, happiness, joy in service; for he that is the greatest among you is the servant of all!   1264-1

Our society seems to have swung to the extreme in bolstering our pride, vanity, and self-importance. There are many schools of thought in popular psychology and New Age factions that encourage us to create idols of our own self-image. Ancient wisdom sends us in the opposite direction—forget yourself, abandon your self-worship, and climb out of that small, confining package of ego. Hopefully, we will eventually understand the teaching that we are here to create happiness and peace for one another first, and as we commit to that, we will in turn receive from others.

Be sincere with self and ye will not be false or insincere with others. The spirit of truth brings the outward appearance of that desire first suggested [the desire to do God's will], if the body and mind are in keeping with that as would be pleasing to the influences or forces called God. For, the declaration of each soul sets in motion that spirit. What spirit do ye entertain? Truth, justice, mercy, love, patience, brotherly kindness? Or self, self-praise, self-glory that ye may be wellspoken of materially? These choices are made by the individual. Their results, their effects in the lives of individuals are such as to determine spiritual success, material success, or a well-rounded mental, spiritual *and* material success. For, the earth is the Lord's and the fullness thereof. The abilities that have been lent thee, keep inviolate— if ye would be in keeping with His purposes with thee.   257-238

"In all thy getting, my son, get understanding." (Prov. 4:7) [Especially understanding] of self. When one understands self, and self's relation to its Maker, the duty to its neighbor, its own duty

> It is more important to know the truth about one's self than to try and find out the truth of heaven and hell.   Hazrat Inayat Khan

to self, it cannot, it will not be false to man, or to its Maker. [Think deeper about this], *for thoughts are deeds,* and are children of the relation[ship] between the mental and the soul . . . What one thinks continually, they become; what one cherishes in their heart and mind they make a part of the pulsation of their heart, through their own blood cells, and build in their own [body], that which its spirit and soul must feed upon, and that with which it will be possessed, when it passes into the realm [beyond the physical plane] . . . The study of these . . . wherein the carnal or material or normal forces are laid aside, and the ever present elements of spirit and soul commune with those of the forces as found in each entity. Study those and *know thyself.*   3744-5

In religious experience one is told *what* to expect, how to expect and when to expect!

In the soul or psychic experience one attunes the God self to the universal [Self]!

Hence the application or experience is from within and in communion with the influence of God-force in the individual life . . .

What is the first thing [to be understood]? *Self!* and the willingness to [surrender] self; willingness to suffer in self . . . for an *ideal!* Not merely idealistic but an ideal that requires first *courage;* the dare to do the impossible.

For with God nothing is impossible, and the individual that may give himself as a channel through which the influences of good may come to others may indeed be guided or shown the way. [Such] influences . . . are those that all men seek, and for which there is a great cry in the earth today—and *today is* the accepted time!

For the harvest is [ripe], but the laborers *are* few!   165-24

And unless each soul entity (and this entity especially) makes the world better, that corner or place of the world a little better, a little bit more hopeful, a little bit more patient, showing a little more of brotherly love, a little more of kindness, a little more of longsuffering—by the very words and deeds of the entity, the life is a failure; especially so far as growth is concerned. Though you gain the whole world, how little ye must think of thyself if ye lose the purpose for which the soul entered this particular sojourn!

Think not more highly of thyself than ye ought to think, yet no one will think more of you than you do of yourself; not in egotism, but in the desire to be of a help. For who is the greatest? He that is the servant of all, he that contributes that which makes each soul glad to be alive, glad to have the opportunity to contribute something to the welfare of his brother. These are thy virtues or thy faults, dependent upon how ye use them.

3420-1

Self–study is a very important aspect of spiritual awakening. We must realize that what is found in a book is a small concern compared to what we can find by studying our dreams and inner world.

8

12 Steps to Enlightenment According to the Cayce Readings

Step 4: Spiritualizing Desires

When the ego's habits have no moral or ethical restraints, our reality is shaped by the lower chakra energies of survival, greed, and appetite. A large part of our addiction to carnal identification comes from an attachment to (1) self-preservation and the fear of death, (2) physical procreative addictions, (3) the desire to control or manipulate others, and (4) accumulation of sensory experiences and material goods. This predicament is exemplified in the Adam and Eve myth, in which spirits discover their ability to physically reproduce and the "knowledge" of sexual pleasure is used for selfish attachments. The "serpent" represents innate spiritual/creative power that is directed downward and externally as sexual activity. It is this reverse flow of the spinal "serpent," referred to in spiritual yoga as *kundalini shakti*, which inhibits enlightenment.

We are faced with a dilemma: do we all have to retain and raise this energy through celibacy? Celibacy is a controversial topic. The Buddha's earliest doctrines were meant for celibate monks and later became adapted for lay people. In ancient Palestine, controversy arose between the apostle Peter and the Hellenized, Pharisaic Jew—Paul (Saul) of Tarsus. Paul insisted that celibacy was the best way to attain higher consciousness, while Peter discounted that idea because never once did Jesus ask him to renounce his wife or family obligations. Jesus accepted Peter just as he was, with family obligations and fiery nature.

Paul tries to walk the fine line between being an idealist and a realist. Although celibacy is his ideal (1 Corinthians, chapter 7), he recommends that people marry instead of being "aflame" with unsatisfied desires. One of the main reasons Paul so vehemently insists on unmarried people and widows remaining single is that he was convinced it was the end of the world—that Christ was returning to take the faithful Christians with him. He states, "The appointed time has been winding up and it has grown very short." (1 Cor. 7:29) Yet two thousand years have passed, and still here we are. So, what to do?

Interestingly enough, the advice of the Buddha and Saint Paul are similar in this way: celibacy frees your mind for a greater focus upon God consciousness if you are trained how. Not only do couples have ongoing marital issues to resolve and manage, but if they have children, their distractions are compounded, leaving potentially less time to focus on God. This is the traditional yogic view: We are here primarily to unveil God consciousness within us, and all other activities are submissive to that principal aim. A couple should be each other's spiritual support, doing what is best for enlightened living. Hence the sages counsel: Let the materialists and apostates do as they wish, without allowing them to influence your dedication to truth (satya).

Once we can transcend the polarity inherent in the recommendation for celibacy, that it is an all-or-nothing proposition, we can see that it is indeed possible to be a sexually active householder and still keep one's spiritual focus. This involves having a partner who is on the same philosophical page as you are, or at least reading from the same chapters. It requires making time for prayer and meditation within the family schedule. It can be manifest as keeping a Sabbath, a day of complete spiritual focus for the entire family.

All of this points to the need for constant evaluation of desires: sexual, monetary, culinary, social, and so forth. Sex just happens to be the strongest biological urge, so it is often stringently addressed by many of the masters. And, as the sages counsel, once you know how to redirect that energy, the various spiritual revelations follow in time.

Some people ask in bewilderment, Why would God give us sex if it was so "bad"? First of all, we gave ourselves the incarnational experiences by moving away in consciousness from God. We are here of our own desire to be independent and to explore the limits of our free will. Second, as carnal animals, we are given the physical ability to procreate, which is a manifestation of the ego's way of keeping carnality in existence. We have used the power of thought to project ourselves into carnal costumes, within the confines of time and space, and here many of us remain oblivious to this predicament. Third, sex itself does not have any moral value; it is merely a biological event found throughout the animal and insect kingdoms. What is "bad" is allowing sexual thoughts to suffocate the subtler ideas of intimacy and kindness, to emphasize the physical act to the detriment of virtue and spiritual union. Again, any time we allow physical phenomena to obscure spiritual truths, we have missed the boat to Christ Consciousness.

For humans, it is the quality of consciousness through which sex is experienced that makes the most impact on a soul level. Lust of any kind creates karma, whether it is applied to greed, violence, dishonesty, or any of the other issues that work themselves into sexual contracts between humans. It is not the sexual act itself that is the pitfall but the dishonesty and violence of an affair; the greed and selfishness of promiscuity; the psychospiritual crisis of pornography. These identify the consciousness through which sexual behavior is manifest, and from the readings' view, it is the consciousness of the individual that is most important in the pursuit of enlightenment. This returns us to the importance of living one's ideal—are you staying faithful to your ideal? If you are, it is not a "sin." If you are not and willingly violate what you know is the right thing to do, it is a significant error and creates karma that must be met.

In the yogic traditions, sexual energy is understood as unmanifest creativity. This primordial energy, residing at the base of the spine, can be externally expressed in sexual activities or internally directed for spiritual communion, what the readings' source commonly calls "attunement." The various sages throughout the centuries have advised aspirants how to redirect these energies. The following activities are some commonly recommended, and effective, methods for redirecting sexual energy:

- Fix the mind on holy, spiritual thoughts (prayers, chants, affirmations).

- Keep good company (stay clear of those that will bring your energetic vibrations down to the lower centers).

- Engage in creative projects (art, music, decorating, writing, etc.).

- Establish an exercise habit (a physical way to transform the energy).

- Keep to a vegetarian diet (animal products are thought to carry ignoble vibrations, the very vibrations that you are looking to transcend). Even if this is for a prescribed period of time, it is helpful in changing one's psychophysiology.

- Live the *yamas* and *niyamas* (all ten of them collaborate to redirect this energy to the higher centers).

- Avoid entertainment with sexually explicit or violent imagery (television, movies, books, music, etc.). The line between sex and violence is very thin, both emanating from the lower spinal centers.

The Cayce source did not recommend that people relinquish all desires but that they commit to spiritualizing them. The difference is that each person is asked to assess a desire based on how it fits with his or her ideal. For example, does this compromise my morality or integrity? Remember, it is the consciousness behind a given desire that is most important to understand.

> The sex impulse is the single most physically magnetic power that pulls the [prana] and consciousness down from the Spirit [in the brain's higher centers] out through the coccygeal center [first chakra] into matter and body consciousness.
> Paramahansa Yogananda

Spiritualizing a desire means getting the ego out of the way and surrendering to Spirit. Spiritualizing sex could mean to see it as a sacred act, symbolic of bringing two sides of Spirit together in an emotionally pure and meaningful union—not being driven by lust or carnal desire but by a centeredness and heart–felt openness that cares for and fosters a devotional connection with the other—where the physical sensations are subjugated to the emotional connection of two people worshiping one Creative Energy.

> For that [misuse of sexual energies] is the source of man's undoing. But [you] who set yourselves as examples in the order of society, education, Christian principles, religious thought, religious ideals, [should] hold . . . to that *love* which is *un*-sexed! [because as a spirit you do not have a sexual/genital capacity.] For He [has] given that in the heavenly state, in the higher forces, there is neither marriage nor giving in marriage; for they are as *one!* Yet [you] say [you] are in the earth, [you] are born with the urge! The [spiritual] awakening, then, must come from within; here a little, there a little. Each soul, each body, that [is committed to Christ Consciousness] as a channel of blessings has received and does receive that within itself which makes for the greater abilities for awakening within the hearts, minds, souls and bodies of the young who question "what will I do with the

biological urge that arises?" *Purify* same in service to Him, in expressions of love; in expressions of the fruits of the spirit, which are: Gentleness, kindness, brotherly love, long-suffering. *These* are the fruits . . . Then [put this in practice] and these [can] become either that which takes hold on hell [self-centeredness] or that which builds to the kingdom within . . .

There are many sex *practices* in the various portions of this land, as in other lands, that should be—*must* be—abolished. *How?* Only through the education of the *young!* Not in their teen age [years], for *then* they are set! When there are activities or speech not explained within the sound or sight of those in their formative years, they, *too*, must one day satisfy that which caused men to come into body-form . . .

Then, by word and by act keep the life *clean!* The urge is inborn, to be sure; but if the purpose of those who [procreate] is only for expressing the beauty and love of the Creative Forces, or God, the [sexual] urge is different with such individuals. Why? It's the law; it's the *law!*   5747-3

The "source of man's undoing" in reading 5747-3 alludes to the readings' recurrent concept of the present state of humanity: spiritual entities that are trapped in carnality (earth–plane consciousness) because of a fascination with procreative powers. Also addressed is the common complaint that we are born with procreative urges—"yet [you] say [you] are in the earth, [you] are born with the urge!" The teaching is this: By raising one's consciousness "here a little, there a little"—with regular prayer and meditation, practicing the seven recommendations for redirecting sexual energies, and living the wisdom of the *yamas* and *niyamas*—one can transcend lust and greed and perceive sexuality with a purified consciousness. It does not necessarily mean that celibacy is mandatory but that we be sexual persons with a spiritualized outlook on sexual intimacy. To spiritualize *anything* means to have spiritual power in control of the material. If higher principles are being trumped by urges or compulsions, the Spirit is not in control.

We have only addressed in detail sexual desire, and yet there is a long list of human desires that can distract the aspirant from God Consciousness—desires that require spiritualizing. The masters recommend increasing one's awareness of desires as the starting place for transformation; you cannot change a poor habit if you are unaware of it. Many people function on a reflexive, habitual level, unaware of what they are doing or why they are doing it. Awareness is just a muscle that too often goes unexercised. If you regularly flex it, you gain more awareness and can catch yourself when you just react or respond without thinking. This is the first place to start to transform desires into spiritual wisdom.

Desire is of a threefold nature [physical, mental, spiritual], and must be controlled only by the mental and the spiritual held as an ideal. 5-2

[T]he mental is *ever* the builder, guided by the spiritual truth and life and light [that] brings for the satisfying of that [built]. Gratifying of selfish influence or desires of self, brings for that as is of the carnal, and makes for dissatisfaction, distrust, dis-ease, in *every* field. 23-1

"For the purpose and intent of Man is to satisfy earthly desires of the flesh rather than that of the manifesting of My Spirit in earth's plane." 139-9

What is spiritualizing desire? Desire that the Lord may use [you] as a channel of blessings to all whom [you] may contact day by day; that there may come in [your] experience whatever is necessary that [you] be cleansed every whit. For, when the soul shines forth in [your] daily walks, in [your] conversation, in [your] thoughts, in [your] meditation, and it is in that realm where the spirit of truth and life may commune with [self] day by day, *then* indeed do [you] spiritualize desire in the earth. 262-65

All desires spring from an exercising of free will. We see chocolate cake, we have a pleasurable sensory memory associated with it, and we exercise our free will to repeat that pleasure. This same delineation basically occurs with the pursuit of every desire. It is a fine line between desire and addiction. All shopping addictions began as standard shopping excursions; all alcohol addictions began as casual drinking; all anger addictions began by self's justification of anger, and often, violence; all gambling problems started as harmless wagering, and so on.

Some people are more prone to addictions than others, yet all of us are addicted to the earth plane—the perpetual cycles of incarnations. The reason why simple living and moral discrimination are such recurring teach-

> It is true that the light of wisdom must continually be kept alight, but it is difficult always to act rightly.
> Hazrat Inayat Khan

ings by the masters is that the more desires and attachments we heap upon ourselves, the more difficult it is to attain the liberation that we yearn for in the deepest level of our spirit.

Spiritualizing desires gives us permission to renounce things that may be unproductive for higher consciousness. It helps us step back and see the big picture of how we are reflexively enmeshed in carnality and removed from metaphysical awareness. Spiritualizing desires keeps the Spirit in the driver's seat of your life, and the ego in the trunk.

9

12 *Steps to Enlightenment According to the Cayce Readings*

Step 5: Increasing Love Through Attunement

An entire lesson (XII) is dedicated to love in Book I of *A Search for God*. In this lesson, coupled with themes recurrent in the readings, a number of important principles regarding love are brought forth relative to spiritual wisdom.

Life itself is the result of the Creator's love for humanity. We have drifted in consciousness from the Source, and the slowed–down experience of the earth plane is the result of a benevolent Creator. As a result of this slower pace, this is the best school in the universe. Yet, with all the inherent distractions of life, it is easy to forget that we are here to spiritually awaken. An important consideration for understanding love from a spiritual perspective is to realize that all creation, the earth and the whole cosmos, was made for mankind's awakening.

The next fact is this: Interpersonal love, when it is pure, takes no inventory. The more self is forgotten, the greater our capacity to love with Christ Consciousness.

What is True Love?

It is not what the romance novels express. According to the readings,

- It is our ability to give and want nothing in return. It is service that takes no account of self's need for reward or reciprocation.
- It naturally prevents us from expressing harsh and unkind words.
- It circumvents the ego's habit of becoming frustrated with people, circumstances, or things.
- It sees all things working together for good, nullifying hate and rancor.
- It fundamentally changes our heart, prompting us to gladly sacrifice for others. This is a natural outgrowth of being closer in consciousness to the Source of all love.
- It breeds empathy, sympathy, and understanding; it holds no grudges of any kind.
- It reveals the truth that "love is God." As one attunes to God consciousness, the Creative Energies are perceived working in and through all people, places, and circumstances.
- It is a consciousness that wholly transcends logical parameters: "My kingdom is not of this world." Jesus; John 18:36 [KJV]

True love is spiritual love. Romantic love is a miniature view of the bigger picture of true love, our deeper need for devotion to the Source. The love of a parent for a child gets us even closer to God-love, but again, this is still a very small dose of it and often still clouded by ego's idiosyncrasies.

He that does not love his worst enemy has not even begun to [spiritually] develop.
"Love," A Search for God

The readings suggest testing ourselves regularly to see just how far we are progressing. One excellent category of testing parameters is our vexers—those who vex us test our connection to God, or to see it another way, our ego immersion.

Many things in our culture get targeted as the object of "love," when in reality it is merely the ego's cravings, or hyperbole. People say they "love" a certain food, but you cannot love food; you desire or crave a food. People say that they "love" a certain type of music, performer, vacation destination, or sensual activity, but in fact they cannot love any of them. As long as the ego is focused on getting something, if cravings are being pursued and expanded, it is not true love. It may be fondness, adoration, the temporary excitement of possession, appreciation, or perhaps titillation, but from the readings' view and the teachings of the yogic masters, it is not genuine love.

> Love is the merchandise which all the world demands; if you store it in your heart, every soul will become your customer. Hazrat Inayat Khan

True love is satisfied with pouring itself out for another, which is a microcosmic vignette for devotion to God. In order to have something to offer in love, a healthy heart and mind, one must be psychologically whole. There is nothing spiritual about supporting unhealthy behaviors. Spiritual yoga focuses on seeing things as they really are—waking up to reality and making the necessary changes in your life that keep you from God consciousness. This is where a good teacher can be valuable. If one is not accessible, then you will have to be fearlessly candid with yourself about your "stuff."

As humans with free will, we are the only species that purposefully moves away from the harmonious way of the universe. All nature (animals, plants, the elements, etc.) is glorifying the Creator and following its inherent purpose, whether or not any of us can directly perceive this connection, especially with our intellectual biases.

Think not that the snail or the dragon fly, as he crawls from his slime, does not glorify his Maker. And as he mounts on his wings of gossamer, he

> The human heart must first be melted, like metal, before it can be molded into a desirable character.
> Hazrat Inayat Khan

fills that place for which he has been—in his realm of activity—designated [created]; in his field, his manner of showing forth his love as manifested from the Creator in the materialized world.

Man alone, of all [God's] kingdom, abuses the gifts that have been made his through the love that the Father would show, in that [man] might be a companion, one with Him; not the whole, yet equal to the whole, able in that realm to magnify, glorify, even as the dragon fly, that love the Father bestowed upon His [children] . . .

Feed, then, upon the fruits of the spirit. Love, hope, joy, mercy, long-suffering, brotherly love, and [divine] contact, the [spiritual] growth, will be seen; and within the consciousness of the *soul* will the awareness come of the personality of the God in thee!   254-68

If we would really get a clear understanding of God's love for us, how patient and forgiving this omnipresent Force is, we have to start changing our hardheartedness. It is useless to wait for some magical time in the future when some great global change is supposed to happen—people have erroneously believed that for at least two millennia. The great change is here and now, making good use of this precious life, if we will only surrender our ego's defenses and submit to God's Way. Many people have found God throughout the ages and there was no stoppage of sociopolitical crises, no magical heavenly brocade falling upon the planet, no shortage of wars and famine, no elimination of all the planetary drama and tragedy intrinsic to this sphere. Amidst all the chaos and turmoil, people have found God by following the ways of the masters—by living the *yamas* and *niyamas* and immersing themselves in *samyama*. It is a personal "second coming," an internal awakening that sees past the drama of the world.

Count it joy, then, even as He, that [you] are called by Him in a service—in a *loving* service—to [your] fellow man; for through this lowly, weak, unworthy channel [Mr. Cayce] has He chosen to speak, for the purposes of this *soul* have been to do good unto his [fellow humans] . . . Love God, eschew evil. Speak oft[en] with [your] brother, [your] Savior, [your] *Christ*, for He is [often in your midst]. He would bless this house, will [you] but keep Him near at hand. Turn Him not away with harsh words, unkind thoughts, or belittling acts one to another! If [you] are faithful to confess [your] faults one to another, He is faithful to forgive; for He alone can purge [your] *soul* and make it light in His *heart* . . . Do good that He may abide with [you], that the clouds of doubt and fear may be purged every whit from [your] experience, from [your] consciousness; and know that He is *alive* in [you], [will you] but love one another even as He has loved you.   254-76

For, all are children and are seeking their way; [often] groping blindly, following those that would lead here or there, when there needs to be the reminding that we must love one another— even as God has loved man and has made manifest that love. And day by day He manifests that love, if those that seek will but open their *heart*s, their eyes, their minds to the wondrous love which God, the Father, has bestowed upon the children of men.
                                                   254-110

When [you] enter into the inner self and approach the throne of grace, mercy, love, hope, is there within self that which would hinder from offering the best or seeking the best from that throne of grace?

Doesn't it then become necessary that such hindrances be first laid aside? even as given of old? When [you bring your] sacrifice, expecting to receive from that throne of grace the mercy and hope desired, [have you] shown mercy? [have you] shown love? [have you] shown consideration in the activities, the associations of each and every individual, whether friend or foe?

Be not impatient with those even that would hinder [you],

from gaining something of this world's pleasures; but know, he [who] seeks to do the biddings of the Creative Forces [God] in a manner that is constructive, gratifies that which is the *soul* development.

For, the soul seeks growth; as Truth, as Life, as Light, *is* in itself. God *is*, and so is life, light, truth, hope, love. And those that abide in same, grow . . .   257-123

Ye may know not God, nor His love, until ye have truly manifested His love to thyself in thy dealings with thy fellowman.
                                                        257-199

Keep the self in such a manner as to be circumspect in [your] own consciousness. Be true to self, making for those activities that bear the fruits of the spirit; just being kind, just being gentle, just being patient, just showing fellowship, just showing brotherly love; just bearing witness in [your] walks, [your] acts, [your] understandings [toward your] fellow man. And [you] shall know Him face to face. For He [has] promised to bring . . . the *remembrances* from the foundations of the earth, of the world, of the universe. For [you existed] in the beginning, even as He.
                                                        261-15

As we try to understand the spiritual teachings from an intellectual level, we often approach God to ask or plead for something. Whether it be a medieval religious view that we are "weak

> *The key to all happiness is the love of God.*   Hazrat Inayat Khan

and lowly" in nature and need God to save us from our "sinfulness" or a New Age view that the universe is a type of great cosmic Santa Claus who has put aside His plans just to give us all the stuff we desire (if we just think the right magical thought combinations), these ego views are erroneous because they focus on taking and possessing. Both strategies are heavily flawed—both are mental barricades to higher consciousness—because they speak primarily to the ego's narrow agenda.

God is your fundamental nature—beyond your mental games, beyond your subconscious scripts, beyond your rebellion, which has formed the illusion of individuality. It is God's Mind which has birthed your mind, God's Spirit which has engineered your spirit, and God's Love which has forged your love. That being the case, you do not need to beg and plead with God—you need to be silent and receptive—you need to be "nonexistent" to truly awaken.

> [The law of love is giving and] . . . is given in this injunction, "Love Thy Neighbor as Thyself." As is given in the injunction, "Love the Lord Thy God with all Thine Heart, Thine Soul and Thine Body . . . " The gift, the giving, with hope of [any] reward or pay is [in] direct opposition of the law of love.   3744-5

10

12 Steps to Enlightenment According to the Cayce Readings

Step 6: Purifying Thoughts

Man may not live by bread alone. Man may not live by the gratifying of appetites in the material world. For man is not made for this world alone. There is a longing for those experiences which the soul, as an [individual] entity, has experienced. And without spirituality the earth is indeed a hell, an individual soul do what it will or may. Such longing may not be gratified from without or in the consciousness of . . . [or experiences of] the forces and influences [outside of] self. For the body is indeed the temple of the living God. Act like it! Keep it clean. Don't desecrate it ever, but keep it such that it may be the place where you would meet [your] own better self, [your] own God-self . . . If [you] would know God, search for Him, for He is within [your] own self! And as [you] express Him in the fruits of spirit; love, grace, mercy, peace, longsuffering, patience, kindness, gentleness; ye will find such within [your]self. . . This is the source of life, the source of love, the source of peace, the source of harmony, and as [you] give expression to same, it may come indeed to [you]. 4082-1

Three areas of moral consternation appear in the teachings as supreme impediments to higher consciousness: lust, greed, and malice. We will address each of them in that order.

Lust: Sexuality and Brahmacharya

When asked in one particular reading if sex was to be used solely for the purpose of physical procreation, Cayce replied:

Not necessarily. These depend, of course, to be sure, on the individual concept of relationships and their activities. To be sure, if the activities are used in creative, spiritual form, there is the less desire for carnal relationship; or, if there is the lack of use of constructive energies, then there is the desire for more of the carnal, physical reaction.   2072-16

In another reading, a forty-one-year-old housewife complained that her husband had been impotent "for many years." She asked if she could have sex with a "trusted friend (a bachelor)" in order to help her "function positively" for the purpose of "carrying on the normal business of home life and work." The reply was a common one for such personal predicaments:

Such questions as these can only be answered in what is thy ideal. Do not have an ideal and not attempt to reach same. There is no condemnation in those who *do* such for helpful forces, but if for personal, selfish gratification, it is sin. 2329-1

This reading returns to a key idea that has been mentioned in various contexts: The consciousness behind sexual activity is the deciding factor as to what is erroneous and what is suitable for a person committed to spiritual living. When there is lust, violence, or any of the morally substandard approaches to sex so common in modern popular culture, the activity will always bring poor results, or "bad karma." When sexual activity is pursued *solely* for the physical pleasure and not for the emotional and spiritual connection with one's partner and with Spirit, then it may be considered problematic. The bottom line is that, culturally, we place far too much emphasis on the physical aspects of sex and very little, if any, on the metaphysical virtues.

> As water is the cleansing and purifying element in the physical world, so love performs the same service on the higher planes.
>
> Hazrat Inayat Khan

Sexuality is an important topic, because all life pivots around it in one way or another. Many of the Buddhist and yogic sutras were directed at monastics, so in those contexts, complete sexual chastity was paramount.

In Asian spiritual traditions, the semen is thought to contain a very powerful energetic essence, one that can contribute to higher spiritual realizations and *siddhis* if it is conserved. Though women are not thought to be as prone to the energetic losses as men, the analogous energetic diminishment for women occurs in successive childbirths, preventing sufficient recovery time—usually at least two years—between pregnancies. In this way, the yogic health traditions declare, a woman's vital energy can be depleted and her energetic reserves insufficient for higher spiritual realizations.

Besides the basic energetic reasons for properly understanding sexual activity, there are psychospiritual ones. The readings' source states that women are innately better sexual stewards because their emotional intelligence trumps their physical urges (unlike most men.) It is when we divorce emotional intimacy and spiritual wisdom from physical pleasure that we have made the gravest psychological error relative to sexuality.

Additionally, keeping one's thoughts on the plane of sexuality confines one's consciousness to the lower spiritual centers. Since sexual and sensory attachments are our oldest vices, they are the most difficult to transcend. There is also a significant connection between endocrine activity and sexual thoughts. It is within the endocrine system that much of the body's karma is stored. The masters tune up their nervous and endocrine systems as the critical inauguration to longevity and God realization. Both the endocrine and nervous systems pay a high price for excesses, reckless sexual choices being a prominent factor.

From a pathological standpoint, endocrine and nervous system diseases are some of the most complex to heal. One considerable reason is that Western medicine still does not acknowledge the existence of the underlying energetic systems of the body. Although great strides have been made in the past ten years, with some Western physicians applauding the preventive benefits of the ancient Asian health systems, there is still a long way to go in transforming our holistically infantile and commercially edacious medical paradigm.

These two physiological systems, hormonal and nervous, are so intimately linked in their functioning that they are often labeled as a singular physiological matrix: the neuroendocrine system. Thoughts, foods, and chemicals all directly affect the neuroendocrine system. Meditation, herbal medicine, Indian *hatha yoga*, and Chinese *chi gong* have been successfully applied for centuries to naturally tune up this complex network.

For neuroendocrine transformation, the core area to start with is thoughts. In a society that uses sex, violence, and greed as its favorite advertising ploys, entertainment plots, and Internet subjects, rising above the cultural din can be challenging. This is where the principles of ancient teachings can be beneficial. The basic recommendation is to (a) avoid violent and sexually exploitive media, (b) keep good spiritual company, and (c) develop strong mental power by magnetizing your consciousness more to spiritual things and less toward carnal ones. This is the essential meaning of *brahmacharya*: one who knows Brahma (God consciousness) by controlling one's mind and vital essence. (For further details on *brahmacharya*, refer to chapter two.)

Sex was not an uncommon subject of the readings. After all, people were conferring with Mr. Cayce regarding real-world issues and were searching for assistance where others had failed them. There were few unyielding moral imperatives when it came to sexual behavior. Commonly, each situation had its own set of subjective parameters—what was "bad" for one person's situation might not be considered so for another. Individuals were prompted to search within themselves for their ideal and how their sexual or emotional behavior corresponded.

Compatibility also had numerous facets—a mixture of past-life- and present-life influences. Mr. Cayce gave a reading for a twenty-one-year-old male in 1928 that hints at the role astrology may play for some in determining compatibility. This young man was told that he had certain proclivities—"Irrespective of will's application"—that he had brought with him into his present incarnation. His reading suggested that, with the proper guidance, he could avoid the potential pitfalls and stay on track with his life purpose. As stated in so many readings, it is *how* one applies one's will that makes all the difference:

> [He is] One that will ever be a student of human nature. Hence in accord with that of the detective, or business, or speaking, or writing. Yet one that may—in an incorrect application of the knowledge or judgment concerning same—bring evil influence in the life; for the entity, while headstrong in many respects, is easily led or persuaded when that as presented—for the moment—represents any desire felt (for the moment) without due consideration given to the fruit of that desired.

So, while he is "headstrong" in some aspects, he is weak in his ability to see the consequences of giving in to a particular desire. Because of planetary influences on his *samskaras* (subliminal tendencies, as they would be known in yoga, which often predict destiny), he is given the following advice:

> Beware of entanglements with those of the opposite sex, especially those whose birthdays come in May. Beware of conditions as pertaining to bodily ills that have to do with the diges-

tive system. Keep self unspotted from low relationships, and
keep thyself bodily clean.   169-1

While he is praised in the reading for having "high mental abilities,"
he is cautioned that his subliminal tendencies are too strong to rely
solely on his mental power. The reading seems to suggest that he has a
natural curiosity about the world in general, which if used for productive ventures would be a positive influence in his life. This same curiosity, though, could get him in big
trouble when it comes to sex. The
reading implies that he will
probably choose the lowest quality option and perhaps contract
a venereal disease. This is what the yogis would call being driven by
one's *samskaras*.

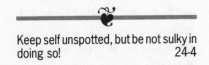

Keep self unspotted, but be not sulky in
doing so!   24-4

Having a strong moral compass, from the readings' counsel, is essential for avoiding the pitfalls of your bad karma. This idea returns in
various forms in the readings: be careful who you "sleep" with, and be
aware of the consciousness through which you engage another sexually. Is it just for physical entertainment, or is it the natural extension of
love, devotion, and commitment? The same could be asked regarding
food: are you eating because you are really hungry or just because you
have nothing better to do? Are you conscious of the quality of the food
you are putting into your body, or are you just carelessly shoveling
something in to fill an emotional void?

Purity of thought is an essential component in the readings and in
yogic traditions. In order to understand ourselves, we are asked to try to
see ourselves as others do, or as the readings state repeatedly, to "stand
aside and watch self pass by."

Greed

This is also the case when it comes to curbing another neurosis: greed.
Lust and greed are intrinsically related—we may even say that they are

two levels of one house of selfishness. Greed takes no consideration of the other person; it always finds a way to justify an erroneous means; it blindly creates many casualties on its way to bolstering its standing. Greed defies the first two *yamas: ahimsa* and *satya*. As if those two "filters" were not enough, there is a *yama* specifically dedicated to addressing this human flaw: *aparigraha*. The tenets of all the world's major religions address greed. It is found in many of the oldest religious parables in various cultures.

> *All that detains man on his journey to the desired goal is temptation.*
> Hazrat Inayat Khan

Yet man in his greed, in his own selfishness, has set himself so [against God's laws] by the very foolishness of his own wisdom.   262-96

> *Temptation, greed, attachment to people and possessions . . . ignorance of your Spirit-nature, idleness, and mechanical living [a going-through-the-motions, thoughtless, robotic lifestyle] are the worst enemies of your happiness.*
> Paramahansa Yogananda[25]

First, look within self. Know as to what is the [motivating] influence within self as to the satisfying of self's own desires, as to that which would maintain the Law of One, of truth, of self within self; or is it—the [motivating] influence [of] avarice, greed, or that which is of self's own desires?   845-1

> *A pure life and a clean conscious are as bread and wine for the soul.*
> Hazrat Inayat Khan

For as He gave, "The heavens and the earth will pass away, but my word—and deed, and kindness and loving thought, *patience*, persistence in the *right* [Truth]—*do not* pass away." They [are] the foundation stones upon which *generations* are [built]. They [are] the foundation stones upon which nations rise that seek to know God. These taken away make for those destructive forces that have arisen and do arise in the experience of nations when man has forsaken God and turned rather to a god of greed, a god of gold, a god of stone, a god of fame, a god of fortune. These fade and die, but the good deeds, the kindnesses, the gentle word [remain] ever.   1159-1

Malice

Better that there be the crust alone of bread than the mansions of the millions with that of a condemning heart, a condemning spirit within self

> *The longing for vengeance is like a craving for poison.*
> Hazrat Inayat Khan

that there is a question mark after any activity, or any associations. For these are not God's ways, and [you have] known and [you do] know in [your] heart of hearts the ways of good! Not that of long-facedness, not that of the saintly sinner, not that of the cynic; but doing good for Good's sake [God's sake], doing good because it brings contentment, it brings harmony, it brings peace, it brings associations that create in the hearts of the associates *joy* and *hope* and the *longing* for the greater knowledge of the *Source* of good. Not just good but *being*, acting, thinking in terms of that honest, due consideration for each and every individual, and not the advantage by chance, not the advantage by foreknowledge, not the advantage in any way or manner over [your] fellow man.

For as in the manner you treat [your] fellow man [you] treat [your] Maker. And [you] *cannot* do that which is [questionable] in [your] own heart and soul [toward your] neighbor . . . wife . . . child, without it bringing turmoil, without it bringing discontent, without it bringing confusion.   417-8

Taking a malicious approach to life situations violates the principal *yama* of *ahimsa*. We may not always be able to emulate the saints, but to paraphrase the Dalai Lama, if we can't be peaceful and helpful in this world, then we should at least not be harmful.

We must be more mindful of what we think daily. We should be very discriminating as to what we allow into our subconscious. In order to spiritualize our consciousness, we must think pure thoughts and eliminate impure ones. We don't have to be perfect, just ever striving for excellence. It is the quality of our inner world that determines the quality of our outer one.

11

12 Steps to Enlightenment According to the Cayce Readings

Step 7: Finding Joy

The readings' source teaches that *true* joy is found not in satisfying self's cravings and desires but instead in the following:

Transcending Ego

Just as the masters teach, the readings counsel that self is the major barrier to interpersonal understanding, spiritual clarity, and oneness with the Universe. It only *seems* that satisfying desires and reveling in passions brings us happiness, but only because we have not experienced the deeper happiness that comes from stepping outside of the ego. When we create enough opportunities to transcend self, we see why the masters and the readings repeatedly teach that ego transcendence is indeed the deeper joy that we seek. There are numerous ways to accomplish this, but the readings emphasize prayer, meditation, and service as the most natural, reliable, and lasting means.

> As each gains, through their own *meditation* or *prayer*, that [they] may be known among men even as they are known with Him, this *takes* on an import. Would [you] act before [your] God in the manner [you] act before [your fellow human]? Love one another. "A new commandment I give, that ye *love* one another." In *this* manner may each see themselves as others see them. Let not [your] words and . . . actions be so different that they are not children of the same family. Let [your] deeds . . . [and] words, be in keeping with that [which] others see in [you].
>
> 262-9

> [The intellect] must turn itself inside out, as it were, see? for it must become *introspective*, rather than outro . . . or extrospective [extroversive], see?
>
> 900-274 [final brackets in original]

> Do not allow the ego of self-praise, self-indulgence, self's fame in any direction, to so override that which is the basic ideal; else we may find this as a millstone rather than a means to those ends in the material, the mental or the spiritual ways being sought.
>
> 257-181

That individuals may of their own volition choose the exaltation of self, or the aggrandizement of self's own ego, is apparent. This makes for

> *The water that washes the heart is the continual running of the love-stream.*   Hazrat Inayat Khan

what many have termed and do term their karmic conditions, [which] may then be seen.

Enter . . . into [your] chamber not made with hands, but eternal; for there He has promised to meet [you]. There alone may [you] meet Him and be guided to those things that will make this life, now, [full of] happiness, joy and understanding.   262-77

Thus may we draw a lesson in our daily experience from this attitude, this condition, this experience [of being on earth] through which each soul finds itself passing . . . The flesh is weak, the spirit is willing.

Will you each as individuals be led by the spirit of truth? or will self, [your] own ego, [your] own material desire, so outweigh that purpose, that hope, that mission for which each soul is given the opportunity in [a physical] expression, that it may be said of you, "except your righteousness exceed the life of the self-righteous, ye shall indeed perish"?   262-125

[Applying yourself to overcome desire] must be realized *within* self. As to how: How would you tell one to fall in love? How would you tell one to apply or make self in accord with God? This *is!* . . . Well, you either do it [by transcending self] or you manifest your *own self!* your *own* ego, your *own* desire!

Make desire, the ego, the self, the whole, as one with—"Not as I will." For how spoke He? "Let this cup pass—if it be Thy Will. Not my will but *Thine* be done in and through me."   264-49

Knowledge is well, and understanding is good; but to use these in a manner in which self—[your] own ego—is to be exalted, makes for confusion to those who would seek to know their place in the activities of the realm of opportunity that is given in the present.   1599-1

Be not overcome with those things that make for discouragements, for *He* will supply the strength. Lean upon the arm of the *Divine* within . . . giving not place to thoughts of vengeance or discouragements. Give not vent to those things that create prejudice. And, most of all, be *unselfish!* For selfishness is sin, before first [your] self, then [your] neighbor and [your] God.
          254-87

All ethics, all human action, and all human thought hang upon [the idea] of unselfishness; the whole ideal of human life can be put into that one word *unselfishness*.   Swami Vivekananda[26]

Surrendering to Spirit

After understanding the necessity for self-transcendence, the next step is to feel in touch with Spirit, living from that joyful, inspired place. Personal whims take a subservient position

Optimism comes from God and pessimism is born of the human mind.
Hazrat inayat Khan

to intuition's guidance and the sublime joy found in serving others. Surrendering to Spirit requires not thinking about, doting on, or protecting self but creating an inner zone in which one is freely guided by faith and virtue.

You then possess true Happiness [if you completely surrender to God and become a channel of blessings to others].
262-111

[F]or that [which] we think upon . . . we become—for "where the treasure is, the heart is also." That which *is* a body's, an entity's ideal, by that the standard of moral, mental and spiritual aptitudes, by that same classification comes the experiences of a

body-consciousness [or an incarnation.] That there are [created] in many [people an] innate prejudice against certain things or conditions, may be oft seen manifest—

When the soul is attuned to God, every action becomes music.
Hazrat Inayat Khan

but the *willingness*, the surrender of self that [one] may be a channel of blessings, not to any [supernatural] source or force . . . but to God! . . . this is the attitude for an entity to take. *Walk* with Him! *Talk* with Him! See *Him* as He manifests in every form of life; for He *is* Life in *all* its manifestations in the earth! and there will [appear] that peace . . . harmony . . . understanding, [which] comes from *humbleness* in *His* name; humbleness of spirit, of mind, of self, that the glories that are [your] own *from* the foundations of the earth may be manifested *in* [you]!   488-6

Put self . . . in the hands, in the mind, of the *divine* from within, and not attempting, not *trying* to be good, [or] kind, [or] thoughtful—but just *be*, and *consecrate* self to the service of others. This peace, this quietness that will come within self from such, will find a ready answer in the mind, in the heart, in the life, in the expression of those—every one—whom [you meet]. *This* is *living* consecration, and not attempting to be moral for moral's sake; not attempting to be good that good may come, but be good that there may be that peace, that understanding, that only comes from putting self in the hands of the divine. Study, then, portions—*any* portion—of the words of Him that gave, . . . "That ye ask in my name, *believing*, that shall ye have within yourself." Do not, then, in asking, make conditions, but surrender self unconditionally into the hands of the divine from within, and that from within shall answer . . . for in Him only is that peace, and the blessings of those whom the body *contacts* will bring the greater joy, the greater happiness. Happiness, then, is not a thing set apart from self, but the conditions [through] which one approaches that in hand to be *done!* for when one considers that the position of self is hard to bear, is not as is desired, the desire of the heart often [makes] one *afraid*—unless that desire is ever in that attitude of "Use me, O God, as I am," . . . He will *not* forsake [you]; neither will He allow [you] to be afraid; for He will raise [you] up, and He understands all the hardships, the *little* things, the separations, the variations in the surroundings—but *trust* Him!

In this manner may the body, the mental body, the physical body, allow the spirit of Truth, peace, joy, understanding, [to] come in and make . . . for self, for those dependent on self, mentally and physically, whole and strong—and able and capable of meeting every issue of every day.   5563-1

So may the entity, with the spirit of God through the power of the Christ Consciousness, come to know—in every thing, in every act—that love [which transcends] all understanding. For, to others it may be as a myth, as a dream, as a thing to be hoped for, but to this body, to this entity, to this soul, who has tasted of the joys of the personal contact with those influences within the soul, it may come to be His power working within.

255-12

Doing for Others

Undoubtedly, this is one of the most recurring themes in Cayce's counseling to others. We are here, having a valuable incarnation, not only to gain personal enlightenment but to serve and care for others along the way, in whatever capacity we can.

Then, today, will [you] not rededicate [yourself], [your] body, [your] soul, to the service of [your] God? And He that came has promised, "When ye ask in my name, that will be given thee in the earth." Then, do not become impatient that [you] are counted . . . as a servant, as an humble worker, as one that is troubled as to food, shelter, or those things that would make [your] temporal surroundings the better. For [you] grow weary in waiting, but the Lord will not tarry; eternity is long, and [so] that [you] may spend it in those things that are joy and peace and harmony, make thy self sure in Him.

> The service of God means that we each work for all.
> Hazrat Inayat Khan

How? "As ye do it unto these, my brethren, ye do it unto me." Just being kind! [Your] destiny is in Him. Are [you] taking Him with [you] in love into [your] associations with [your] fellow man,

or [are you] seeking [your] *own* glorification, exaltation, or . . .
fame, or that [you] may even be well-spoken of? When [you] do,
[you] shut Him away.   262-77

Loving thy Neighbor (As You Wish to be Loved)

This takes the previous concept one step further. One's neighbor is
not just another who looks like you, thinks like you, speaks your same
language, or shares your same racial genomes . . . but *everyone*. It is not
enough to tolerate your neighbor—even your enemy—but we are counseled to love others, forgive them, and extend endless compassion. This
is a tall order, a highly challenging one to do consistently, and yet it is
the essential foundation of Christ Consciousness. It goes against everything with which the ego feels comfortable, which is a good clue that it
has spiritual power and veracity. Once we really feel that everyone is a
part of our family and treat one another with the same care and concern, we are on the way to higher consciousness.

12

12 *Steps to Enlightenment According to the Cayce Readings*

Step 8: Living a Balanced Life

Another principal lesson from the yogic masters and the readings' source is the idea of keeping balanced in all things. Practicing moderation is paramount to good physical and mental health. One cannot invest in one's physical self to the detriment of one's emotional or intellectual self. Physical activity, intellectual development, healthy emotional expression, and a common-sense diet are all to be well balanced. Of course, what makes this tricky for any individual is either (a) not cultivating the ability to be honest with oneself, (b) refusing good counsel, (c) allowing rebellion to intercept the messages from one's common sense and intuition, (d) allowing oneself to be an extremist in one or more areas and have addictions, or (e) some combination of the above.

There needs to be precautions as to the [right] physical activity

[and] diet . . . that the body [better] budget its time, its activities. Not only should there be mental and physical labors, but mental and physical relaxations, mental and physical improvements, mental and physical recreations of those natures that are in keeping with a well-rounded life and experience . . .

Budget the time, the activity, so as to keep a well balanced life experience in *all phases* of its mental and physical activity. All work and no play is [counterproductive], or all relaxation without sufficient activity for the full strengthening of the body. Either of these may be taken to extremes. But take the time for the work, for the play, for recreation, for improvement in *every* activity or manner—these are [recommendations] that keep a body well balanced . . .

Play, work, activity of every sort that requires the use of the body is the better. At times a great deal of walking, at times being in the water, at times *any* form of exercise that does not *overtax* but that gives the muscular activities needed for the body. All of these should be a part of the experience.   257-225

The following reading is at par with the masters' teachings, that mere satisfaction with life is not the authentic goal of an incarnation. The goal of life is a complete and uninterrupted connection to higher consciousness—full enlightenment—to know God's will and be living completely in accord with that, with no traces of ego impeding or diluting that connection. This is a lofty goal indeed but in accord with best teachings.

All work and no play will destroy the best of abilities . . . The life must be a well balanced life, not lopsided in any manner, to bring contentment—not necessarily be satisfied, for that is to become stagnant; but . . . in whatever position [you find yourself], force self to be *content* but *not* satisfied, knowing that the applications of the spiritual, mental, and physical laws are but the pattern one of another, and in so setting self in this direction all must be working in coordination and cooperation . . . 349-6

The next reading alludes to the fact that slow, steady progress is the best method of advancement in the spiritual life. Instead of striving to be a huge bonfire, we are encouraged to be hot coals, intense with the desire for God's love and guidance and patiently staying aflame for the long haul . . . as many lives as it may take. The reference to being "defeated" acknowledges that we are here to overcome challenges. The spirit of the message here is more likely akin to *he that* seems *defeated but overcomes through persistency, consistency, and intuitive wisdom.*

> [There is] the *opportunity* of self in the [present] experience to not go to the *extreme* . . . But keeping self well-balanced in all things . . . will bring those [circumstances] that make for the greater development in the experience of a soul. For [it is not] the extremist [who] excels, but rather he that is often called the plodder, he that is often defeated—but not defeated in the *soul* purposefulness of that whereunto self has set self to a task in the material things of life.   361-4

Having a moderate and natural approach to life is the consistent recommendation in the readings. The whole point is to life live with an intuitive guidance that is being deepened daily through the practice of meditation.

> [Questions such as] What shall I read? [With what] shall I be clothed? Where shall I dwell? What shall I eat? and the like, become the questions of many. He that [takes] thought of such has *already* limited the powers that influence through those forces in life. The *natural* things . . . are the things that make for the better physical body in normal activity. *Normalcy*, not extreme in any manner! and there will be shown [to you] day by day that which will be . . . necessary for [your] *own* development. To some [a] certain amount of exercise, certain amounts of rest, certain amounts of various characters of breathing, of purification, of prayer, of reading—as is found necessary; but [above] *all* be true to that [you promise] that source from which all health, all aid, must come!   5752-2

The next reading may be summarized with the following: the less that ego leads you, the fewer mistakes will greet you.

> Study to show thyself approved unto *God*, a workman not ashamed, rightly dividing the words of truth, keeping self unspotted from the world, keeping self unregenerated in that there are no making of experiences for which the body will be sorry. For remember, it is self meeting self.   257-166

An important component of living the balanced life is seeing the world through optimistic "glasses." You will have to get through your karma one way or another—you might as well choose the positive, optimistic path.

> Keep optimistic, and keep spiritually balanced. For the sources of mental and material influences must arise, as so oft has been given, from a spiritual import that is *constructive!* Hence an individual that does not *think* constructively builds barriers to be tumbled over sooner or later.   261-25

> [K]eep the mind balanced, as to what each is to do! Expect something, and something will happen! Do not expect anything and most anything *may* happen!   255-3

Some people erroneously think that being spiritual means living an uninformed or sequestered-from-reality existence. We are all called to be of service, and only by staying aware of where service or healing is needed can we answer our calling.

> The secret of life is balance, and the absence of balance is life's destruction.   Hazrat Inayat Khan

If we use the body as an analogy, we may get a clearer understanding of the intention of the following reading. It is small pain signals that alert our nervous system to an imbalance. If we ignore the small pain signals, the body, in its infinite wisdom, sends bigger pain signals to motivate us to action—to making a change in the status quo. Dis-ease occurs by repeatedly ignoring the wisdom of the body—its many calls to action. We are each like the white blood cells of the immune system, called to preserve the health of the organism (our community and planet), which we do by taking action through service, prayer, and spiritualized intention.

> Keep self well-balanced, and keep the body physically fit, the mental body alert, and the spiritual body—give it an opportunity to manifest . . .
>
> As [for] the spiritual life of the individual, this may be termed one life while the material activities may be termed another. But, if they are not made to coordinate *throughout*—and that preached in one direction and not lived in the activities, then—sooner or later—one or the other must bring destructive forces. Do not become a crank on any subject! Do not allow self to be led entirely astray, but keep self well-balanced in the material activities, the mental activities and mental abilities, acquainting self with what is *going on* in the material world, the mental world, the social world, and using same—not altogether for self's *advantage*, but that the body may be, in its abilities in every sense, the better able to serve and manifest—through the activities of self—that it would worship in its inner shrine.   342-1

Balance is the keynote of spiritual attainment.   Hazrat Inayat Khan

Three areas of balance are addressed by the masters in various ways. We can delineate them in the following manner.

Physical

- Do not overeat—one should finish a meal feeling just a little unsatiated.
- One should eat real foods—not ones processed, packaged, or perverted from their original form. Eat more organic whole grains, fruits, and vegetables.

- Get the right amount of sleep. Too little puts a person in a state of sleep deprivation, creating an increased inability to effectively manage stress as well as a tendency to gain weight. Too much sleep dulls the mind and reduces energy levels. Eight hours is usually a sufficient amount for most people. The more one attunes to Spirit in deep states of meditation, the greater the neuroendocrine changes in the body and, naturally, the less sleep is needed.

- Exercise the body daily. From a yogic viewpoint, this does not necessarily mean performing a cardiovascular aerobic exertion as much as practicing yoga *asanas*, which build strength and flexibility in the muscles and joints and compress the major glands that lie anterior to the spine. The point is to increase *prana* (breath/energy) in the spine and tissues, not to just raise the heartbeat to some theoretical rate.

- Stay clear of intoxicants—not just the obvious culprits of alcohol and recreational drugs but also chemicals found in cosmetics, cleaners, and packaged foods. Much has been reported in the popular press about the health benefits of drinking wine. What is underreported is that the same basic benefits can be achieved by drinking pure, unsweetened, unfiltered grape juice. The latter is just as beneficial as the former in its antioxidant benefits. Taking drugs—as alcohol, hallucinogens, amphetamines, narcotics, and the like—is the easy way out to a deep-seated need for an alteration of consciousness. We have within our psyche the distant memory of God consciousness, and to rely on drugs for an experience

> *There can be no better sign of spiritual development than control over passion and anger. If one can control these, one can control life.*
> *Hazrat Inayat Khan*

of altered consciousness is a lazy means to try to reconnect with that. It is best to transform one's consciousness through spiritual practice—to get high on God. This is the real "high" that we are all seeking, whether we consciously realize it or not.

Mental

- Meditate daily. This is the most organic method to reorganize brain-wave functioning and improve mental abilities.
- Manage your stress well. We may not be able to eliminate stressors, but we always have a choice in *how* we choose to respond to them. If the ways that you have learned are not working for you, learn some new ones.
- Find more ways to laugh. As long as you are not enjoying another's misery or suffering, which would annul the *yama* of *ahimsa*, enjoy as many opportunities to laugh as you can. Laughing helps boost your immune system naturally. And it is found that happy, jovial people are statistically healthier people.
- Be an optimist. The adage *see the best, expect the best, work for the best* is an ideal way to frame your reality. Optimism helps one see new opportunities as well as create them.

Spiritual

- Meditate daily. Besides providing important mental benefits, this is the single most potent activity to bring one's ego consciousness into a greater awareness of God consciousness. The only people you will ever hear that detract from the powerful transformative benefits of meditation are those who do not regularly and deeply meditate.
- Pray—not as a beggar or a menial subordinate, but as a child of the Most Divine. Pray not just to receive things from God but to change yourself, to transform your learned selfishness into selflessness. Pray for others: those who struggle more than you, those who have less than you, those who suffer more than you, those who are further from God in consciousness. Pray as an act of co-creation with Eternal Spirit.

13

12 Steps to Enlightenment According to the Cayce Readings

Step 9: Patience

In the readings, patience is addressed on many levels—each being emphasized as essential to spiritual advancement or maturity. The cardinal teaching about patience is that it is seeing life from a soul viewpoint. When seen outside the ego's tiny lens, life can be understood through patience. From a soul's view, closer to God's view, the path to enlightenment is a long road, and we must work diligently to do God's will.

The readings repeatedly emphasize patience as an important spiritual view on life. There are three main areas of patience to consider: (1) As we work to aid others, putting aside our selfish desires, we get a clearer understanding of the meaning of spiritual patience; (2) As we refrain from retaliating against others, turning instead to Christ Consciousness within, we use patience as an active force to transform our ego habits; and (3) As we stop pretending that we know God's Way through our intellectual strategies, we can legitimately enter into Higher Consciousness. This is active patience with ego surrender.

The first level is the path of karma yoga—working wholeheartedly to serve others. All teachers and caregivers know the precious value of patience. *Maybe we are not all called to be patient with one another* is the sentiment of some people who seek to take the easy way out. Of course, such individuals have been on the receiving end of someone's impatience and missed a great opportunity to see themselves. We all seek, even expect, others to be patient with us—but do we extend the same unconditionally to others? The first lesson in patience asks us to try this.

> [A]s patience is learned, and selflessness, more and more there may come peace and harmony by the very thought, the very act, the very influences the entity may bring to bear in the experiences of others.   2247-1

> For, though ye gain the whole world in *every* way of fortune, fame or what not, and lose hold of that love that cometh from just being kind and patient, ye have lost that harmony, that peace which comes from being at one with [Christ Consciousness].   262-121

> Be ye faithful; even as ye would have mercy show mercy; as ye would have peace give peace; as ye would have patience shown [to you] be patient with others; for only in the attributes *of* the living forces of God may ye *find* God; *not* in the *material* things that make of earth-earthy gratifications!   294-136

The following reading was counsel to a twenty-two-year-old female. This advice was given at the end of her reading, concerning the ideal mind-set for a physical healing, probably the one area in which, more than any other, people sought help from Mr. Cayce.

> Go slow; or make haste slowly. Be patient with self and with others. Do not work self into a state of overanxiety at the

changes that will be found, or attempt to use up the strength and vitality mentally and physically to gain or maintain those balances that once were held [in the body]; for these will come in their normal time. Forget not the source of thine inspiration in self, for they must be in the God of life, of truth, of hope, of love.   480-11

The next level of patience is to refrain from retaliating, or attacking those who attack you first. This is in alignment with the teachings of the *yamas*. We can dislike someone's behavior, knowing that it is coming from the illusory trash heap of the ego, and still hold respect for that person's spirit. The readings say that to control or redirect anger is better than having no temper at all. Emotions are potential energy and it depends on *how* we direct that energy that makes for a plus or minus mark upon our spiritual general ledger. It is always easier to redirect energy than to try to create something from nothing.

One that may control self in anger is beginning the first lessons or laws of experience. One that may control self in anger, that must come as resentment [caused by the words of others], may make for that which disregards the words said; disliking that which would produce such a feeling within self, yet able to love the soul of one that causes or produces such a state of feeling [in yourself]. This is patience, and love, and hope, and meekness, and pureness of heart . . .

Then with patience wait for that awakening which will make for an understanding of that necessary to overcome—even as He. Taking stock, then, with self, one may know whether it is patience, faith, virtue, knowledge, brotherly love, or what, lacking in self. Do not find the fault in the other, but rather cleanse thine *own* mind, heart and soul, and the proper attitude toward whatever problem that presents itself will be in that manner of understanding love that knows no fear, but being content in *His* praise, His love, His understanding.   262-25

The readings counsel people
to extend patience toward them–
selves. For some, it is easy to be
patient with others yet far more
difficult to be patient with one's

*Lack of patience starves virtue to
death.   Hazrat Inayat Khan*

own learning process. As the masters repeatedly teach, we can understand another only to the depth that we understand self.

> For few there be who comprehend that if they are patient first
> with their *own* selves they are then more capable of being, more
> able to be, patient with others.   1158-2

Both the masters and the readings agree on this one tenet: God's
ways and man's ways are rarely the same. We often seek out a winner
and a loser in a conflict. God does not; God seeks victory for all. We
often think that there must be one right way or method, while God has
created many. We judge by appearances and intellectual data, while
God looks upon the heart and soul of an individual. It is having the
wisdom to take this macrocosmic view that helps breed patience.

> This is then the Wisdom that is shown in the life, in the experi-
> ence of each soul. It is through the variations, through those
> activities that make for the thinking, the analyzing, the seeking
> for God and God's Wisdom, that man is brought to the closer
> understanding; making for that consciousness within the expe-
> rience of each soul that in patience, in long-suffering in broth-
> erly love, is Wisdom. Yet as judged by man in the earth . . . [this
> is often perceived as] weakness. But the weakness of man is
> the Wisdom of God. Just as the knowledge of God, the Wisdom
> of God applied in the daily experience of individuals, becomes
> strength, power, beauty, love, harmony, grace, patience, and
> those things that—in the lives of those who are applying same—
> make for a life experience that is worthwhile, even in the tur-
> moils of the earth and those activities of sin and sorrow and
> shame and want and degradation . . .   262-104

The following excerpt is an example of a recurring theme in the readings: It is not enough to wish someone well; we must *do* something to "aid . . . comfort . . . or cheer." If you have a broken leg and cannot fend for yourself, it is useless for another to *think* you a glass of water; an action must be taken on your behalf. Having helpful thoughts is the first half of the equation, but without helpful actions, it is an incomplete and faulty spiritual recipe. The readings' view on patience is that it *must* be active, not passive.

> Keep in that way, in patience, in persistence, in sincerity, in truth. [Do not falter when] there are periods when apparently little is seen to be accomplished externally. Know that [you have] set in motion that leaven that [works metaphysically], yet will bring the consciousness of His love, His hope, His presence, into the lives of all. Each should be patient first with self, in honor preferring one another. Sit not in the seat of the scornful. Stand not in the place of the cynic. Be mindful not of things of high estate; rather give place to that that makes for sweetening in the lives of all; for he that wishes his brother well, yet makes no move to aid or supply, or to comfort, or to cheer, is only fooling self. He that would know the way [God consciousness] must be oft in prayer, joyous *prayer, knowing* He [gives] life to as many as seek in sincerity to be the channel of blessing to someone; for "Inasmuch as ye did a kindness, a holy word, a clothing in act as to one of these the least of my little ones, ye have done it unto me." As He [knows you], so may [you] know Him, [you] who have been chosen for the various channels of activity in spirit, in mind, in body, for the manifesting of His glory in the earth. Be faithful. Do not allow self to be so overcome in *any* manner as to miss that calling in Him; for He is faithful who has promised to be near.   281-12

From the view of the readings' source, active patience is a kind of *tapas*—a discipline that helps refine the sharp, jagged edges of the ego into a smooth, useable surface. This person asked how she could be "less sensitive and more adaptable":

> Just be that way! that is, as this: Do not worry self [about] conditions that have so long existed where the [mind and body have] depended upon outside influences for abilities of activity. Then, as the conditions are physically and mentally adjusting themselves, just be patient with self and with others. The more patience that is shown in self toward others, the more patience will be shown by others to self—and it becomes then a circle, as it were, and before one knows it the conditions have adjusted themselves so that the self is able to adapt self to all the circumstances and conditions, and the environs that come about in the various activities. Being patient . . . with self first, being patient then with others. As the patience is manifest, so will the results be seen. This doesn't mean patience in the sense of just submissiveness, or just being quiet—but an *active* patience, *conscious* of being patient with self and with others. Force self to do some unpleasant things that it hasn't wanted to do once in a while, and like it!   911-3

> But the *greater* development may come not in [criticism of others] but in . . . constructive aid to individuals *struggling* to know what is constructive in their experience. For this, then, would make for those experiences when the little niceties—that are the natural tend[ency] of the entity—become selfless and more for the advancing of the activities of others . . . [F]or he that would have life must give it; he that would know God must be—in the attributes of the earth—in those things that are of the spirit: Gentle, kind, longsuffering, brotherly love, and—most of all must this entity learn—patience! That the entity has fallen in oft . . .
>   [Patience is not withdrawing or fleeing] . . . This is not patience, for patience is [neither] passive nor negative; it is a *constructive* influence, a positive activative force. For, if one smite thee on the one cheek, did He say withdraw? No! Rather, turn

the other! Be active in thy patience; be active in thy relationships with thy fellow man! . . .

Remain not on the outside [in externalities]. Have patience first with self; then look within. For thy body is indeed the temple of the living God, that is within thee. When thou fearest from those things from without, then look within—and there ye shall find comfort and joy and harmony.   815-2

In the urge arising from these influences we find that there is the necessity for the entity to learn a little more of Patience. For Selfishness is not a portion of the entity's own being; rather is it the lack of the Patience; not with others but the more with self. For as He gave, it is in patience that [you] become aware of [your] soul!

So in its associations with others the entity needs to forget those things that have made for hardships, . . . for misunderstandings in relationships . . . whether with individuals or with groups; though the entity may find oft that it requires that self turn within, that the consciousness of His Presence abiding may direct. Thus may there be brought peace and patience, as an *active* force; not as a passive influence in the experience of self but as an *active* influence!

This has brought into self that association where tolerance has not *always* been felt, as may be seen through the appearances [akashic record of reincarnations] of the entity in the earth; not tolerance as a passive thing but tolerance as an active force! . . . [Know] that each soul is destined to become a portion again of the First Cause, or back to its Maker. And as there is the awareness of its individuality, its ability to apply its portion, the *soul*-portion of the Creative Forces or Energies or God within itself, it builds that in a soul-body which may be One with that Creative Force.

Keep that faith [you] *innately* [have] in the *oneness* of power in the Creative Forces as it makes for manifestations in the hearts and minds of men; and as [you] do it in [your] activities with [your] fellow man, as [you] do it in [your] meditation, as [you] do it in [your] mind, so will it be meted to [you] in [your] inner self . . . So must [you] temper [your] judgements . . . [and] find [your] patience . . . For if [you] would have mercy [you] must show mercy to [your] fellow man; yea to [your] very enemy, to those that despitefully use you. Laugh with those who laugh; mourn with those who mourn, in the Lord. *Keep* [your] paths straight, and [you] will find *glory—glory*—unto [yourself]!

987-2

Learn again patience, yet persistent patience, active patience— not merely passive. Patience does not mean merely waiting, but as it does for those that would induce nature to comply with nature's laws. So with patience, comply with patience's laws, working together with love, purpose, faith, hope, charity; giving expression to these in thy daily associations with those ye meet; making thy daily problems as real as real life-experiences, pur- poseful in every way.   1968-5

14

12 Steps to Enlightenment According to the Cayce Readings

Step 10: Service

As we read in step 7, "Finding Joy," service is a means to transcend the self, and in transcending self, we find great joy. The Cayce source is emphatic that this is an essential component of living Christ Consciousness and the true measure of a person's spiritual realization:

> [I]n service alone may any soul find advancement or development . . .
>
> 721-1

Heaven, the Cayce source and the masters clearly state, is a state of consciousness—the result of how you are mentally programmed and how you live your life here and now. Our heaven consciousness is intrinsically linked with helping others: "You'll not be in heaven if you're not leaning on the arm of someone you have helped." (3352-1)

Just as Master Yeshua (Jesus) had to return in the body to rec-tify his karmic debts, so too must we understand our challenges as karmic lessons in need of our at-tention. The Cayce source stated

The one who wants to become a master must first pass through an examination as a servant.
Hazrat Inayat Khan

that making one's consciousness at par with the Christ nullifies karmic debt. Service helps one transcend selfishness and move closer to Spirit, to rely on a Higher Power to work through the body–mind for the good of another. Selfishness and karma are two sides of the same metaphoric coin.

> *Practice* . . . charity to all, love to all; finding fault with none; being patient with all, showing brotherly love and brotherly kind-ness. Against these there *is* no law [or karma]!   1620-1

Patience is required (as step 9 states) as we forge ahead and do what little we can to serve our community:

> Don't be weary in welldoing. If it requires years, give years . . .
>   3684-1

The great yogis also emphasize the need to serve others. We are asked to simultaneously develop ourselves and serve others. If done well, they both reinforce each other:

> It is more pleasing to God if you work consciously for Him, rather than for yourself. If one works in the world, and cares only for self and family, it is much more difficult to expand beyond the confines of ego-consciousness. Wise is he who views all human-ity as his own greater family.   Paramahansa Yogananda[27]

The readings state that each soul has taken an incarnation to find God, whether one's personality is aware of it or not. Of equal impor-tance is our mandate to take care of one another. We are all created from the same Source as spiritual siblings, and a large part of spiritual maturity is realizing that we cannot hate a fellow human and love God.

[W]ithout service to the other, one may gain little in *this* experience in life's forces, for Life itself *is* a service.   53-1

[S]ervice to others is the highest service to the Creative Energy [God].   69-1

All knowledge is to be used in the manner that will give help and assistance to others, and the desire is that the laws of the Creator be manifested in the physical world . . . All power is given through knowledge and understanding. Do not abuse that power lest it turns again and rends the perpetrator of such conditions . . . For God is Spirit and they that worship Him must worship in spirit and in truth and, as has been made manifest in the flesh, with all power, all knowledge . . . [M]an must overcome through the knowledge [of Christ Consciousness]. The last to be overcome is death, and the knowledge of life is the knowledge of death. See? Any who may seek knowledge is seeking the greatest gifts of the gods of the universe, and in using such knowledge to worship God renders a service to fellow man. For, as given, the greatest service to God is service to his creatures . . .
                                                                  254-17

One of the unfortunate byproducts of the New Age movement is the usage of spiritual ideas to bolster the ego's desires. There have been numerous movements centered on teaching individuals that they can have whatever they want; they just need to want it intensely enough. If the ego is not purified in advance of this pursuit, then the result will be accumulating wealth, power, and goods to the detriment of one's soul wisdom. If a particular approach insults the spirit of the *yamas* or *niyamas*, know that it is erroneous. One cannot defy the *yamas* or *niyamas* and expect to eventually prosper on a spiritual level. Both the masters and the Cayce source clearly warn against cheapening the ideal for material or personal expediency:

Then the ideal in the material: An opportunity to serve all, or opportunity to rule someone else? Remembering, he who would be the greater will be the servant of them all.

    The ideal, then, of the material: Is it plenty of money, or position? Or the opportunity to use that [which you have] in hand for the glory of the God, for the benefit of [your] brother, for making the world where [you] are a better place to live? For, if [you] are a "taker" and never a "giver", what have [you] accomplished?

5253-1

God cannot escape you if you catch Him in the net of divine meditation and divine service. One of these without the other, however, is spiritually dangerous. You need the balance.

Paramahansa Yogananda.[28]

Yogananda clarifies this by stating that meditation alone may cause a person to become too withdrawn; and service alone, without consistent meditation, causes a person to rely on his ego too much, forgetting his reliance on Spirit. But by balancing the two, "Then work helps your meditation, and meditation helps your work. You need the balance."[29]

There are many ways to serve, and each person must take inventory on how to best use his or her gifts. For some, it is working with people—spending time with an elder who is isolated and lonely, serving children, assisting in hospitals or hospice facilities, or aiding the developmentally disabled or infirm. For others, their efforts of service are called to nature—

[Have] *over all* that mind which was the mind of Christ-Jesus—service to man, that all may know the face of God.

294-71

working in animal clinics, cleaning trails or beaches, volunteering with the forest service or district parks, starting or maintaining community gardens, and so on. Some have skills in building or in construction management from which a group or community would love to benefit. Others find fulfillment in combining these service opportunities, expanding the scope of their opportunities to be a "channel of blessings to others." All who have served from the heart know the great and sublime joy that comes as a result. After experiencing this, then, the meaning of this chapter dawns upon the individual: As one transcends self through serving others, one moves one step closer to God consciousness.

In cooperation *is* the offering of self to be a channel of activity, of thought; for as line upon line, precept upon precept, comes so does it come through the giving of self; for he that would have life must *give* life, they that would have love must show themselves lovely, they that would have friends must be friendly, they that would have cooperation *must* cooperate by the giving of self *to* that as is to be accomplished—whether in the bringing of light to others, bringing of strength, health, understanding, these are one *in* Him.   262-3

In this age, in this period when there are the doubts, the fears, those seekings for expression in all the many and varied ways, it will be [wise] to keep the balance; . . . [for balance ensures] the greater advancement, [and] a sureness of self in its daily efforts. While [it is fine to experience all the beauties of life, we are called to serve one another daily. Service must be an everyday personal duty that brings inner fulfillment.] For we grow in grace, in knowledge, in understanding *from within*. And even though there are the words of the mouth, even the activities of the body, if they are done, if they are *meditated* upon to be seen [by others], to be feeling, to be making only an outward show, these must eventually come to naught. For the *kingdom* is within. Contentment, peace, harmony, glory, love, beauty, is from *within*; and . . . that which will bring the growth, the understanding, the environments, the necessary influences. For with all the labors, the efforts, with all the application of beauty, of strength, of power, of might, *only* God may give the increase.

165-21

15

12 Steps to Enlightenment According to the Cayce Readings

Step 11: Embracing Challenges

It is important to remember that we are primarily here to grow spiritually, not to bask in creature comforts or sensory pleasures. The challenges in our life are opportunities to understand ourselves on a deeper level. The idea of *santosha* prompts us to accept our present karmic lot as the perfect circumstances for our spiritual development.

The *niyama* of *tapas* helps develop our inner strength. Being able to accept things that "burn" us, that compel us beyond our comfort zone and force us to rely on our innate metaphysical power, is essential to appreciating the gift of *tapas*.

The readings' source reveals that for many, "war with the infinite within" is the result of a lack of "stamina, faith, patience or what not." (2174-3) For many people, a significant challenge they face is being able to sit quietly and meditate daily. Time and again the readings' source counsels people that the answer they seek externally can be found—and *should* be found—within, if they would just do the work in attuning themselves to Spirit in prayer and meditation. This is *tapas*: to overcome one's restlessness in order to find the sublime joy of introspection.

The readings' source promotes the veracity of numerous biblical metaphors, largely because Mr. Cayce's conscious mind was most familiar with them and they provided familiar axioms for the people seeking readings. The emblem of fire was used numerous times as a teaching metaphor, the biblical *tapas*: "But know, each and every soul is tried so as by fire; purified, purged; for He. . . learned obedience through the things which he suffered." (281-16)

This idea of being purged as a prerequisite for enlightenment is a recurring theme in the readings and the yogic traditions. *Tapas* is the events and circumstances which purge one of selfishness, of ego consciousness. In the readings, there are essentially two choices that a person makes with any dilemma: do you satisfy self or do you glorify Spirit? Just as many of the masters teach, pain is the greatest spiritual teacher, the one thing that brings people to God more than anything else. This being so, the readings convey the difficult truth that suffering is the most efficient way to refine the ego: "[T]hrough trials, trouble, tribulations, one arrives at the best things in life, and trials are forgotten." (288-1) Of course, this is true only if the suffering expedites ego surrender and not rebellion.

Both the readings and the masters' teachings emphasize the fact that pain in this world is a remarkable teacher:

> The man who is groping [his way] through sin, through misery, the man who is choosing the path through hell, will [eventually] reach freedom, but it will take [a long time]. We cannot help him [more than he wishes to help himself.] Some hard knocks on his head [experiencing pain and suffering] will make him turn to the Lord. The path of virtue, purity, unselfishness [and] spirituality, he will know at last, and what he has been doing unconsciously [searching for pleasure] he will do consciously [searching for enlightenment].   Swami Vivekananda[30]

This world is a realm of continuous dichotomies. What is commonly exalted by those of material consciousness is shunned by the mystic and spiritual master.

> A diamond must be cut before its light can shine out.
> Hazrat Inayat Khan

The treasures of the materialist are a bane to the sages.

When one is suffering, it is an opportunity to surrender to Spirit and turn one's consciousness toward the metaphysical. When we, as spiritual aspirants, encounter others who are suffering, it is an opportunity for us to serve them—to comfort and enlighten them in whatever way we can. This is what the readings' source refers to as "bearing the cross of others." The "cross" is analogous to karma, and as we meet our karma, working through our selfishness and spiritual rebellion, the "crown" is the eventual result—enlightened consciousness. We are not to take others' crosses from them, robbing them of their opportunity for soul growth, but we can help them bear the weight by sharing the "crowns" of compassion and wisdom.

For philosophical materialists, those bewitched by material luxuries or content with a life consumed with the perpetual pursuit of endless desires, their spiritual fulfillment is delayed by the misuse of their free will. The reason that every soul has taken an incarnation, the readings' source states repeatedly, is to discover God as a living Reality. Within that scope, everything that supports this goal is grace, and everything that distracts from this goal is "sin." What the world exalts as desirable or acceptable—lust, greed, malice, laziness, revenge, and so on—is seen as repugnant from a spiritual view. In many instances, incarnating in a distressed body or within a troubled environment is an outstanding growth opportunity for a soul, even though such a person is pitied by most people. Although, on a soul level, entities do choose this, it should never be a justification for us not to serve them in their distress. For, just as they choose a challenging circumstance as their ideal karmic "medicine," we too choose to encounter them and are then given the opportunity to help relieve their suffering. This is the way of Christ Consciousness. For anyone to dismiss such suffering as "just their karma" and not do anything to help allay their hardship is disgraceful and completely antithetical to spiritual wisdom.

The proper understanding of *tapas* (purposeful suffering) and the "cross and crown" may evade many students of metaphysical or religious thought. For some in orthodox Christianity, this idea is oversimplified as *Jesus died for my sins, and in believing in Him, I am saved.* For many embracing New Age beliefs, the idea of *tapas* is shunned in favor of consulting an external oracle for some kind of insider shortcut: a channeler, tarot card reader, crystals, and so forth. In both of these belief systems, soul transformation is avoided by reliance on some external "it"—a church's manmade creed or a channeler's limited ideology, for example. Both the readings' source and the masters counsel that the "church" is first and foremost within. In the inner church there is the opportunity to enter into the "holy of holies," or the sacred spot between the eyes (the eye of wisdom), and attune directly to the Source of consciousness. Neither the pastor nor the channeler can ever do your spiritual work for you. And in the overall rubric of the masters' way and the readings' source, what you believe is subordinate to what you do, how you treat others, and what choices you make daily. These three activities, done well, determine spiritual competency.

The payoff of spiritual attunement through prayer and meditation, and the cumulative effect of *tapas*, is a greater surrender to Spirit and a feeling of love. The challenges we face, however, need to be properly contextualized. If they are not, it is easy to feel overwhelmed or even defeated by life's disturbances. What is created in the earth plane must be met in the earth plane, and that is why we are here:

> [D]oubts and fears and desires and disturbances . . . burn and burn, yet all must be tried so as by fire. And the fires of the flesh in their activity in material associations must be purified in . . . love . . .   294-174

The readings' source states in numerous ways that one's karma is annulled by at–onement with Christ Consciousness.

A common worry by some is that one is expected to be karmically flawless before enlightenment dawns. But this is not the real way of things. Christ Consciousness is a daily awareness of Spirit working through people and nature, of a joyous heart calling to its transcendental Parent, and of applying just a little more patience, kindness, understanding, and wisdom—to others *and* ourselves. Christ Consciousness is the first-rate means to enlightenment, and it requires that we accept *tapas* as a critical step to an expanded consciousness.

> *Whether a small-minded person loves you or hates you, in either case he will pull you down to his own level.*   Hazrat Inayat Khan

16

12 Steps to Enlightenment According to the Cayce Readings

Step 12: Deep Meditation as the Path of the Masters

Samyama is the path of the mystics. It is turning within in a whole-hearted and devoted manner and discovering unparalleled transformative spiritual dimensions. *Samyama* breeds Christ Consciousness. According to the great yogi Paramahansa Yogananda,

> The stages of enlightenment are, first, to be conscious of the AUM vibration throughout the body. Next, one's consciousness becomes identified with that AUM vibration beyond his body, and gradually throughout the universe. One then becomes conscious of the Christ consciousness within the AUM vibration— first in the physical body then gradually in the whole universe. When you achieve oneness with that vibrationless consciousness everywhere, you have attained Christ consciousness.[31]

Yogananda is describing the process of achieving enlightenment, from the beginning stage of *pratyahara* to the advanced stage of *samadhi*. A natural aid in pursuing this spiritual progression is a deeper attunement to the AUM—the ever-present sound of Creation and the vital energy within and through all life. Both the yogic masters and the readings' source repeatedly refer to the transformative power of attuning to the AUM.

In the yogic tradition, the sacred spinal energy is sometimes known as the *kundalini shakti*. It is the upward movement of this spinal energy as the organic result of consistent spiritual practice, which breeds God consciousness. The readings sometimes refer to it as the "I Am" within. Both attuning to the AUM vibration and opening the heart center affect the raising of this sacred energy.

In correctly attuning with the AUM, it is important to recognize that we are not singing—this is not a performance hymn. The sound is internal, meant to vibrate the glandular structures and awaken the *kundalini shakti*, or the internal "I Am" in the spine. One should take the sound within, feeling one's cranial bones or throat region vibrate.

> Let the deeper self, the real self, enter into the deep meditation that the I AM consciousness may make [one] more and more aware of how the purposefulness of the [present life] may be applicable . . . This is most [desirable.]
>
> 649-2

> These as they may be sounded within; not just the vocal box of the physical but as they rise along the centers from the bodily forces to unite the [neuroendocrine] activities . . .   1770-2

The readings suggest that attuning with the AUM even facilitates physical healing, or as in most cases, attunement itself is the prerequisite for physical healing. (1861-12) It is critical to remember that one meditates not to get something from it, not even a healing, but to know/realize God within; physical healing is the natural result of this realization:

You [meditate] because you desire to be attuned with Creative Forces [God energies]. You don't [meditate] because it's a duty or because you want to feel better, but to attune self to the infinite!
                                                               1861-18

In order for true healing to occur, there has to be an inner awakening—some kind of internal shift. It is our connection to the metaphysical Light and Love that we call God which brings about the greatest changes:

[A]ll healing—of every nature—*must* come from the spiritual. It is the attuning of same to the divine within self that brings healing forces.
                        1861-11

As ye open thy consciousness to the Great Consciousness within, there will arise more and more the white light.
                                                   987-4

Some people become overly analytical as to what pitch they should be toning AUM. Some will even play bells or bowls and think that the power is in the physical implements. It is not. What is most influential is not the pitch of the note or the external device but the intensity of devotion and focus of the mind and heart. This has *far* greater power than external devices. If this is well understood, external devices can be employed by meditators in the beginning as temporary assistance. If this is not well understood, it is best to just tone AUM by itself and practice withdrawing the mind from sensory habits.

The tone, then—find it in thyself, if ye would be enlightened. To give the tune or tone [a particular note or pitch] would mean little; unless there is the comprehending, the understanding of that to which ye are attempting to attune—in the spiritual, the mental, the material.
                                                   2072-10

Many aspects of the 281-13 reading have been presented so far, but it is worthwhile to recap the information given in this reading on medita-

tion. It has elements reflective of the yogic teachings but remains idio-
syncratic in the way the readings' source presented the mystic arts.

"Meditation . . . is prayer from *within* the *inner* self, and partakes not
only of the physical inner man but the soul that is aroused by the spirit
of man from within." Deep meditation, *samyama*, is the process of getting
connected to our soul awareness. There is a physical/energetic change
that occurs as the result of "the shutting out of thought pertaining to
activities or attributes of the carnal forces of man." This is why so much
emphasis is placed, in the yogic traditions and in the previous chapters,
on transcending desires. As our mind releases its intense grip on carnal
desires, issues emanating from the lower three chakra centers, it frees
up an enormous amount of energy to be used for returning to Enlightened Mind.

We are told to set an ideal and move into that. The readings are
biased toward the Christ Light as is found between the eyebrows, in the
area some call the "third eye." It is left to the individual to assess whether
a cleansing—some type of purification ritual that is meaningful to the
aspirant—is necessary prior to meditation.

We are reminded that "healing of every kind and nature" can occur
as the result of the concerted focusing of thought. Even today in hospitals throughout China, people are taught meditation to focus the power
of their minds on their own healing. Entering meditation with "a clean
body, a clean mind" can help us "receive that strength and power" as
appropriate to each person.

All this and more is possible in meditation as we enter into the stillness and silence and merge our consciousness into the AUM, or the
eternal sound of God.

[In Patanjali's Yoga Sutras] *Aum* is spoken of as the symbol of
Isvara or God . . . Further, Patañjali says that deep concentration on *Aum* is a means of liberation . . . The scriptures classify
ordinary chanting as (1) repeated loud utterances of the word
Aum, (2) repetitions of *Aum* in whispers, and (3) continuous
chanting of *Aum* in one's mind, listening to it mentally.
Superconscious chanting, however, is that in which the mind is

> deeply directed to the repetition of, and the actual profound
> listening to, the Cosmic Sound as it vibrates in the ether. This is
> the true way of contacting God as he is expressed in creation
> . . . the real or superconscious chanting of Aum . . . consists not
> in an imitative vocalization of Aum, but in actually hearing the
> Holy Sound.   Paramahansa Yogananda[32]

The previous exposition and all the information throughout this book on meditation and Christ Consciousness are intended to inform the spiritual aspirant. The truth is, you need just a little information to start meditating. Reading about advanced stages of realization is in many ways an impediment because it presents experiences that are not yet yours. It is better to get busy creating the introspective habit, and let the meditations teach you about the rest.

Meditation is the process of stripping away one's poor mental habits, born of spiritual rebelliousness. You are not gaining anything by meditating; you are undoing, unraveling, and unfettering self-created delusion. The less expectation you have, the better; the less you try to conjure up some experience, the better.

One of the many valuable contributions the sacred teachings of India have given the world is the power of meditation to reveal God. God cannot be found in a book. If that were not true, the world's librarians and scholars would be the holiest sages of all, not to mention the countless lawyers and law clerks. Books inform us, sometimes even misinform, but appeal primarily to the intellect. Reading is a good way to nourish the mind, perhaps elicit emotions, but attaining God consciousness requires that we step way beyond that level and seek within for a more profound and lasting understanding of who we are as Divine creations.

This does not discount the way in which sacred texts are worshiped by many religious cultures. What they are really in reverence to is the lineage of important teachers that penned their inspirations and passed them down for others to benefit. This is how God works through people. But it is crucial to understand what a text represents and not become bibliophile idolaters. All sacred texts should prompt the aspirant into action—to change one's bad habits and cultivate good ones, to turn within in a greater way, to surrender to God, and to serve and love all humanity. It is the precious human spirit that is most valuable—most worthy of adoration. As a meditator, you get authentic experiences of your soul self and have something internal to rely on.

The following are some teachings on various meditation approaches. Just as in all art forms, there are many ways to achieve a good result. The following paragraphs are from teachers who each have a provocative view of the mountain. Hopefully, this will inspire you to start climbing.

> Meditation is sticking to one thought. That single thought keeps away other thoughts. Distraction of mind is a sign of weakness. By constant meditation it gains strength, that is to say, the weakness of fugitive thought gives place to the enduring background free from thought. This expanse devoid of thought is the Self. Mind in [its purest state] is the Self.   Sri Ramana Maharshi[33]

> To be spiritual is not to be an angel with wings, but something infinitely greater—one who is in touch with God. You must live differently than the ordinary [person], who is in touch only with sense consciousness. Spiritual consciousness lies in absolute victory over human consciousness. Now, spirituality does not mean only to meditate; it embraces a very wide field of controlled existence [yamas and niyamas, for example]. However, meditation is the best foundation. It is the greatest way to be spiritual, the simplest way to spiritualize the consciousness . . . but to meditate, on the one side, and be angry or lead a desultory life on the other, is like putting your feet in two boats going in opposite directions. You must not only learn to meditate, but also learn to behave. To have spiritual consciousness is to be able to do those things that are in your highest interest. And I can bet that ninety-nine percent of the people do not know in what lies their own good.   Paramahansa Yogananda[34]

Meditation is luminosity. It illumines our heart. When illumination takes place in our heart, insecurity and the sense of want disappear. At that time we sing the song of inseparable oneness with the Universal Consciousness and Transcendental Consciousness. When our heart is illumined, the finite in us enters into the Infinite and becomes the Infinite itself. The bondage of millennia leaves us, and the freedom of infinite Truth and Light welcome us.   Sri Chinmoy[35]

The culmination of *samyama* is the manifestation of Christ Consciousness. As the readings and the masters' teachings declare, productively applying yourself in society is an important responsibility of higher consciousness. There are many ways to effectively accomplish this. The readings repetitively emphasize serving those in need, meeting each person at his or her own level of understanding. We may use any of the following terms interchangeably: *nirvana, samadhi, kensho, enlightenment,* or *Christ Consciousness.* The following section explores some of the readings related to the preferred term in the readings, *Christ Consciousness.*

The Christ Consciousness is a universal consciousness of the Father Spirit. The Jesus consciousness is that [which] man builds as body worship.   5749-4

Readings Relative to Christ Consciousness

Reading 262–14

(Q) Is the faith of man in Buddha or Mohammed equal in the effect on his soul to the faith in Jesus Christ?
(A) As He gave, he that [receives] a prophet in the *name* of a prophet *receives* the prophet's reward, or that *ability* that that individual spiritual force *may* manifest in the life of that individual. Hence, as each teacher, minister or seer, or prophet, receives that obeisance as is giving the life from that faith and hope as held by . . . an individual . . . [who] approaches [in] that

> manner [of losing individuality or ego consciousness] . . . Hence,
> as we find, each in their respective spheres are but stepping-
> stones to that that may awaken in the individual the knowledge
> of the Son in their lives.

Translation: All paths are valid as long as they afford you the opportunity to lose sight of self and experience Spirit as a living reality within.

Reading 262–70

> Let that desire, that thought, that purpose, be in each of you
> that was in the *man* Jesus that, though He were in the world yet
> not of the world, neither was He strange nor curious, neither did
> He [refrain] from partaking of those things that were about Him
> in the social, in the home life of His fellow man. Yet His desire
> [was] ever, "Not my will but Thine, O Lord, be done in me.

Translation: Jesus did not make himself stand out in public by being
strange or odd in any way but actively engaged people in whatever
sphere of activity he met them, no matter how seemingly mundane. His
main objective in life was to be a channel of God and inspire all those
whom he contacted.

Reading 272–9

> Then, just being kind, just being patient, just showing love for
> thy fellow man; *that* is the manner in which an individual works
> *at* becoming aware of the consciousness of the Christ Spirit.

Translation: True spiritual development is not measured in your psychic abilities, extrasensory perception, or telekinesis but rather in your
ability to be consistently patient, kind, and loving—*those* are the most
impressive powers you can bring to the world.

Reading 436–2

[S]tudy—through that known in self of the spiritual and mental forces active in [your present incarnation]—to show [your]self approved unto an ideal that is set . . . in the Christ, knowing that in possessing the consciousness of His love, His manifestation, all is well; for, as is known, without that love as He manifested among men, nothing can, nothing did, nothing will come into consciousness of matter. Not that we may deny evil and banish it, but supplanting and rooting out evil in [your] experience, replacing same with the love that is in the consciousness of the . . . Christ, we may do all things in His name; and using those opportunities in whatsoever . . . activity the entity may find to show forth those commands He gave, "If ye love me, keep my commandments." What, [you] ask, are His commandments? "A new commandment give I unto you, that ye love one another." What, then, are the fruits of love? The fruits of the spirit; which are kindness, hope, fellowship, brotherly love, friendship, patience; these are the fruits of the spirit; these are the commands of Him that [you] manifest then in whatsoever place [you] find yourself, and your soul shall grow in grace, in knowledge, in understanding, and that joy that comes with a perfect knowledge in Him brings the joys of earth, the joys of the mental mind, or joys of the spheres, and the *glory* of the Father in [your] experience.

Translation: Evil exists as a manifestation of the unrefined ego, and this can be transformed by realizing the Christ Mind, which entails practicing the fruits of the spirit—kindness, hope, fellowship, brotherly love, friendship, and patience. The "spiritual fruits" bring lasting joy.

Reading 440–4

[The fruits of true spiritual development] may not be measured in or by the ways of the finite forces, or the finite mind, but

rather they are measured by the consciousness of the spirit
. . . in the life and in the experience of Jesus, the Christ, who
thought it not robbery to make himself equal with God, yet found
himself of no estate; rather enjoying the experiences of his [fel-
low man] in every walk of life, and using those experiences in
such a way and manner that [nothing derogatory] could be said
of the life of the man, and [nothing] could be said in the experiences of those that knew Him best, other than "He went about
doing good."

Translation: Do not rely on the opinions and whims of spiritual rebels
and philosophical materialists to gauge your spiritual development.
Become one with God in meditation while humbling yourself in greater
ways; spend your days going about "doing good" for others. If the igno-
rant deride you for being a do–gooder, take that as a great compliment,
as Jesus was a do–gooder, and know that one day, they will need someone to serve them as well.

Reading 410–2

For, truly does the soul live on and become . . . more and more
aware of that which is done in an unselfish manner, so that it
may become more and more aware of abiding and living and
being in Christ Consciousness. And hence the greater *soul* development . . . for any *soul* is to be less and less of self, less
and less with *material* desire, but more and more in accord with
the Christ, the Holy One, the Life, the Manifestation of all those
things that have been said to be so impractical as related to
materiality; yet they are the *real*, the *true* things in the experiences of every soul. Woe is he indeed that may hold a grudge,
or that may build upon those things that are termed hardships
in his experience! Rather, as He, rejoice in the crosses that [you]
may bear with Him as [your] aid; then indeed does that compan-
ionship become such as to make for those joys in [your] daily
life in such ways and manners that [you] see the fruits of the

spirit of the Christ manifested in the lives and *hearts* of those to whom [you] may be only gentle or kind in the passing. For, did not the poet give, "He smiled and the whole day was bright"? The song came, and the cheery word came to another, and the load was lifted from those that had thought [they had] a burden too heavy to bear. Just being kind and gentle, just being patient and giving in the experiences with those one contacts day by day, brings that joy, that pleasure, that understanding, that can *only* come with walking with Him. And He is very near unto [you]; He is in [your] own heart, [your] own life, day by day.

Translation: Some people may say to you that expanding your spirituality is impractical or not as important as gaining material things, but do not listen to them. Challenges, disappointments, or painful episodes are an opportunity to surrender to Spirit and purify the ego self. The more you are connected to Spirit, the more will greater joy and inner delight infuse your mind, the more will you have patience and understanding with people and events.

Reading 538–30

[Be] more constant [in] meditation . . . putting into action day by day a little more patience, a little more love, a little more forgiving, a little more prayer. These *develop* the mental of the subconscious to that point of *spiritual* activity. Being made in the flesh, heir to the weaknesses of same, one becomes more spiritual by the even balance that is obtained by making *personal* application [of spiritual ideals] . . . even though it [may] hurt . . . [to do] that [which] will aid another; *not* that self is to be crucified [so] that another may have *ease* in the material sense. That another may have *understanding* in the mental and *spiritual* sense, sure; for "my yoke is easy, my burden is light" is *seldom* understood. When the desire and the purpose [and] application [are] one—then it becomes easy; but when they are at variance one to another, hard *is* the way, and the call of the flesh becomes strong.

Translation: The more you meditate, the more you tune your conscious mind to the subconscious. This in turn allows you to refine the effectiveness of your intuitive compass, which will afford you more patience, love, and forgiveness. Sometimes you will be asked to serve another to the point of it being uncomfortable to your ego—that is the time to surrender to a Higher Power. When you are guided by Spirit, all will work out well.

Reading 452–7

(Q) Is the Roman Catholic Church the true Church founded by Jesus Christ through the Apostles?
(A) This would depend upon who was asking for such. As we would give here, the *church* as founded by Jesus Christ was, is, the catholic [universal] church but *not* the *Roman* Catholic Church! This has rather been added, as have most of those—in their activities—that call or classify themselves as churches. For, the true church is within you, as the Master, as the *Christ* gave himself: "I to *you* am the bridegroom—I to *you* am the church. The kingdom is within *you!*" Hence that which has been coordinated into the bodies in any activity [is a] representation *of* that which has gathered together for coordinating activity in whatever field; but are most man made. [author's underline]

Translation: The real church always has been, always will be, within your own consciousness.

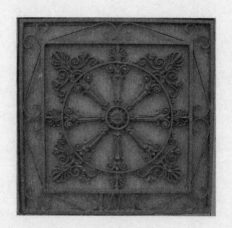

Chakra

17

The Forgotten Years of Jesus, Yogi Extraordinaire

It is exceptionally odd that seventeen years of Jesus' life are missing from the Gospels and that modern Christianity as a whole seems highly unconcerned about this enigma. Why would Matthew and Luke go into painstaking detail about his genealogy only to omit seventeen of the most formative years of the *Messiach* (Hebrew for Messiah, meaning the "anointed one")?

In Luke's story, Jesus is taken to Jerusalem for his bar mitzvah and is lost for three days, which in itself is quite curious. When he is finally found, he is in the temple "sitting among the teachers, listening to them and asking them questions." (Luke 2:46) Then chapter two ends with Jesus' family returning to Nazareth with him. The subsequent seventeen missing years are accounted for with, "And Jesus increased in wisdom and in stature and years, and in favor with God and man." (Luke 3:52) Chapter three has Jesus being "about thirty years of age" when he starts his Palestinian mission, the missing biographical section seemingly irrelevant to the writer. (Luke 3:23) I call this the Christian version of the Nixon tapes—seventeen years gone in a flash—the status quo highly unconcerned and no one left to account for it.

The readings help complete important sections of this historical gap. And fortunately, someone did ask in a reading the following question:

Q. Why does not the Bible tell of Jesus' education, or are there manuscripts now on earth that will give these missing details to be found soon?
A. There are some that have been forged manuscripts. All of those that existed were destroyed—that is, the originals—with the activities in Alexandria.   2067-7

Of course, we want to know *how* he increased in "wisdom and stature." Just what was he doing for that time? Knowing the critical biographical information of Jesus' travels lends understanding to this aspect of his life, widening the scope of his influence and presenting him as a much more transcultural figure than is traditional.

The readings' source affirms that Jesus was an Essene, as was his whole family, including his cousin John the Baptist and John's family, although "John [the Baptist] was more the Essene than Jesus. For Jesus held rather to the spirit of the law, and John to the letter of same." (2067-11) This would be an important role Jesus would play and exemplifies for all of us the necessity to hold rather to the spirit of a teaching than to mere manmade dogma. This is the enlightened approach.

Six important facts emerge in the readings about the historical Jesus relative to his role as a *mahayogi* (*maha* meaning "great," and *yogi* meaning "one who is yoked"):

1. His primary teacher was a woman (which would influence his progressive cultural attitude toward women.)
2. He was an Essene, although still very much a mystic.
3. He traveled through Persia, India, and Egypt, spending the majority of his life as an expatriate.
4. He did *not* have romantic relations with Mary Magdalene.
5. He had a great sense of humor, often laughing and joking (just how many traditional pictures have you seen representing Jesus smiling or laughing?).
6. He had twenty-nine lives previous to his last—at least six as key figures in the development of Judaism and the Jewish Bible, and as a soul, influencing *all* philosophies of monotheism.

Jesus' Teacher: Judy the Essene Priestess

One of the leaders of the Palestinian Essenes was a mystical priestess named Judy. The Essenes apparently had a liberal church leadership policy, allowing both genders to serve equally as leaders and teachers. Judy was influenced by many cultural religious philosophies:

> [W]e find the entity [Judy] came in contact with the Medes, the Persians, the Indian influence of authority—because of the commercial association as well as the influence that had been upon the world by those activities of Saneid [a teacher from India] and those that were known during the periods of Brahma and Buddha.   1472-3

If Judy indeed knew about Vedic and Buddhist philosophy and she was the teacher of Jesus, it would be logical that Jesus was familiar with it as well. This could be one reason why Jesus' words appear so Asian in philosophical tone in the Gospel of Thomas, the important Gnostic text discovered in 1945. Some people consider the Gospel of Thomas to be closest to the original sayings of Jesus—single-line quotes outside a narrative context.

Judy's story is a complex one. The readings state that both her parents and their religious community expected a son and were quite disappointed when her mother delivered a daughter:

> That the entity was a daughter, rather than being a male, brought some disturbance, some confusion in the minds of many.   1472-3

Apparently, the community members and leaders had received spiritual messages that they would be gifted with an important leader with the new birth. Many were dumbfounded that it was a female child. This, the readings state, would be an omen that women were to be honored as spiritual powers, equal to men. Jesus would take this awareness with him and defy convention by openly teaching women and making them leadership equals with the males.

(Q) Why was Judy not a boy as expected?
(A) That is from the powers on high, and gave the first demonstration of woman's place in the affairs and associations of man. For, as [with] the teachings of Jesus, [this] released woman from that bondage to which she had been held since the ideas of man conceived from the fall of Eve, or of her first acceptance of the opinions—these were the first, and those activities that brought about, in the teachings materially, that as Jesus proclaimed.   2067-11

So the message in brief is that women were to be regarded with a higher socioreligious stature. Jesus taught that men and women were equals, which would have contradicted the rather misogynistic Semitic traditions of the Middle East. Even today, the remnants of this antiquated ideology—that women are innately inferior to men—can be seen in the scarcity of female leaders in religions worldwide. Whether it be the Catholic bishops, Jewish rabbis, or Muslim imams, women are still not institutionally regarded as viable religious teachers. Even the Buddhists have very few females as leaders. In many Buddhist countries, it is still not culturally acceptable for women to be monastics; being a leader of a monastery is an even greater challenge. There are a few notable exceptions in the world, and it will mark the beginning of a *real* New Age when women emerge as equals in political and religious leadership. We are currently seeing on the world stage the struggle between the old patriarchal paradigm and the new equanimity paradigm.

Judy was an example of how a woman could be an intellectual, a scribe, a teacher, and a mystic. The fact that she disappeared into anonymity should not be a major surprise, based on the cultural influences of the times.

According to the readings, she was also very human and not celibate. Jewish tradition does not necessarily hold celibacy as a paragon of religiosity. Rabbis are encouraged to marry, so it would seem apropos that a female teacher would do so as well.

The readings do not expand on Judy's personality much, except to say that she had quarrels with some of the community members. There are also conflicting details about her age at both the time of Jesus' birth and his death. When the readings' source was queried as to why there are no records of the existence of Judy the Essene, the answer was simply that the Essene records were not valued by Palestinian society as much as were the Jewish and Greco-Roman. Even the Samaritans, who were looked upon with great disdain by the Israelites, had better chances of culturally preserving their traditions than did the Essenes. This was likely due to the secretive nature of the Essene meetings and the high degree of misinformation which that promoted. We could even speculate that religious bigotry was an influence, especially since the Essenes gave women so much authority.

Contrary to cultural concerns of the era and much to the surprise and delight of her parents, Judy became an astute apprentice of the religious and mystical traditions. She would familiarize herself with the religious ideas of Persia, India, Egypt, and even Buddhism.

> Hence not only the manners of the recording but also the traditions of Egypt, the traditions from India, the conditions and traditions from many of the Persian lands and from many of the borders about same, became a part of the studies and the seeking of the entity Judy early in the attempts to make, keep and preserve such records. 1472-3

She was "the prophetess, the healer, the writer, the recorder—for [many] groups" that were associated with the Essenes' activities and, later, Jesus' life. (1472-1) This must have been quite a revelation for the fifty-seven-year-old radio program producer who came to Mr. Cayce in 1937, while he was giving readings in David Kahn's home in Scarsdale, New York. During her first reading, the magnitude of that revelation does not seem to have even registered. She was a teacher of Jesus and one of the chief leaders of the Essenes! And yet she came with normal problems and questions, just like everyone else seeking guidance from the readings' source. It seems that because of her sensitive nature, she was suffering from physical problems and depression. The Cayce source also chastised her a bit in her reading for being careless regarding her health.

As Judy, she apparently lived to be ninety-one years old and func-

tioned as one of the most important scribes of the Palestinian Essene
community. She was also quite spiritually attuned:

> Here we find there had been, for the mother of Martha, an expe-
> rience of coming in touch with Judy who had been the first of
> women appointed as the head of the Essenes group who had
> the experience of having voices, as well as those which would
> be called in the present experiences communications with the
> influences which had been a part of man's experience from the
> beginning, such that the divine within man heard the experiences
> of those forces [externally] and communicated in voices, in
> dreams, in signs and symbols which had become a portion of
> the experience.   3175-3

The following dialogue gives us a little more insight into her later
years and her exceptional abilities:

> (Q) Was she present at any of the healings or the feeding of the
> multitudes?
> (A) Those where she chose to, but she was very old then. She
> lived to be sufficiently old to know, of course, of the feeding of
> the first five thousand. She was present, but rather as one that
> brought the crowds together, than as contributing to the activi-
> ties at the time. For, there the divisions arose, to be sure.
> (Q) Was Judy present at the Crucifixion or the Resurrection?
> (A) No. In spirit—that is, in mind—present. For, remember,
> Judy's experience at that time was such that she might be
> present in many places without the physical body being there!
>   2067-11

The yogic traditions of India have long worshiped God in the female
form—goddesses hold a special place in the Hindu henotheistic view.
Having a female teacher familiar with Indian philosophy, coupled with
his own experience of living in India for years, would predispose Jesus
to the divinity of women. It was before women that Jesus would lan-

guish on the cross, and it was to women that Jesus would first appear after his physical metamorphosis.

The Ancient Essenes

The Essenes were established by Samuel during the time of Elijah and "were students of what ye would call astrology, numerology, phrenology, and those phases of that study of the return of individuals—or reincarnation." (5749-8) The readings state that the Essenes were at odds with the Sadducees because the latter did not believe in reincarnation. Even back then, this topic was controversial, as it remains today in many orthodox sects.

The disciples must have had some understanding of the concept of reincarnation when, in Matthew 17, they ask,

> Then why do the scribes say that first Elijah must come [before the Messiach can appear]?
> He replied, . . . Elijah has come already, and they did not know or recognize him, but did to him as they liked . . .
> Then the disciples understood that He spoke to them about John the Baptist.   Matthew 17:10-13 [author's brackets]

The historical Elijah would have been dead a few hundred years by the time that question was asked. Certainly, they knew that the spirit previously known as Elijah had returned in the physical as John—else that question would have been nonsensical.

> Because of the divisions that had arisen among the peoples into sects, as the Pharisee, the Sadducee and their divisions, there had arisen the Essenes that had cherished not merely the conditions that had come as word of mouth [oral tradition] but had kept the records of the periods when individuals had been visited with the supernatural or out of the ordinary experiences; whether in dreams, visions, voices, or what not that had been and were felt by these students of the customs, of the law, of

the activities throughout the experiences of this peculiar
people—the promises and the many ways these had been interpreted by those to whom the preservation of same had been
committed.   1472-3

The Essenes were mystics who kept records of their traditions and
experiences. They had an oral and written tradition, spanning back to
the time of Melchizedek (a previous life of Jesus), of supernatural or
spiritual experiences of their people. Being raised in an Essene environment, Jesus would have been keenly aware of these experiences as well
as the law of reincarnation.

The Essenes were a group of individuals sincere in their purpose, and yet not orthodox [according to the view of] the rabbis
of that particular period. Thus [the nature of their gatherings]
would be described by the meditations, certain ritualistic formulas, as may be outlined . . . from the activities of the priest in the
early period when there was the establishing of the tabernacle.

Remember, recall, the first two [temples] didn't do so well,
even under the direction of the high priest; for they offered
strange fire.

Let not, then, that as would be offered here [in the present],
become as strange fire, but as in keeping with the precept of
Jesus, "I and the Father are one;" not individually, but in the
personal application of the tenets, commandments, being one
in purpose, one in application.

Thus [an Essene] meeting would be [for] the interpreting of
each promise that has been made; as to when, as to how there
would come the Promised One.

Analyze in the mind, then, that from the 3rd of Genesis
through to the last even of Malachi. Set them aside. Use them
as the basis of discussions, as the various groups may be set in
order; each rotating as a teacher, as an instructor for that
particular meeting; remembering all [the Essene meetings] were
secret meetings.   2067-11

The likely meaning of the term *strange fire* is reminiscent of what the yogis call "yogic heat." This is when the *kundalini* energy is forced to rise too quickly in the spinal canal and the spiritual centers are affected too intensely, causing physical and even mental distress. Two common media that create this unwanted result are hallucinogenic substances and forced breathing exercises. Both of these methods are shunned by the spiritual masters as being inorganic shortcuts that lead to detrimental results.

Some people in India have been committed to asylums because of yogic heat. Because the Western medical models do not yet accept or understand energetic and *kundalini* phenomena, the orthodox treatment a victim of yogic heat would receive could never address the central problem. Only a yogic master and healer would be able to potentially remedy this complex problem, and even then, there would be no guarantees. The yogic masters know very well that you do not play around with "strange fire."

What cultural anthropologists and archaeologists know of the Essenes is still very scant. Even with the discovery of the Dead Sea Scrolls, it seems that there were multiple sects of the Essenes, all of which had variances on how they implemented their beliefs. It was once thought that the Essenes were strictly reclusive communities, but further studies have revealed that they were well incorporated into many cities as well as having sequestered communities in remote areas.

It is not much different than metaphysical groups today. If two thousand years from now people are trying to understand just what today's "Metaphysical New Agers" thought, the ultimate answer would reveal that beliefs and creeds varied widely from region to region and group to group. Although there may be sequestered metaphysical communities here and there, the majority of people with an interest in metaphysical spirituality are well incorporated into communities all over the world. The Essenes were basically in this same boat, just in their particular historical context. It is well to keep in mind that the Dead Sea Scrolls, which some erroneously think definitive of the Essenes, represent only a few facets of their religious philosophy.

It should be remembered that Essenes were Nazarenes, the translation of which from Hebrew means "branch." The Nazarenes were branches, or offshoots, of the Judaic tree. The Bible records that early Christians were called Nazarenes, signifying that they were Jews who, while remaining faithful to many Jewish activities and traditions, believed in Yeshua's (Jesus') messianic role. They were fully Jewish, but as an offshoot of the orthodox systems.

The Essenes focused on mysticism and self-purification as a path to create the right environment for the long-awaited Jewish Messiach. Jesus fulfilled that role primarily because he, as a soul, was responsible for the subsequent waves of incarnations in the earth plane—according to the readings' source.

Principally through his previous incarnations as Enoch, Melchizedek, and Asaph, Jesus was personally involved in the lineage that helped comprise the Essene tradition. The incarnations of Jesus, as revealed in the readings, divulge a missing link to the greatness of this soul. Understanding his involvement with humanity's incarnational event, as well as the fundamentals of Judeo-Christian thought, explains this entity's true archetypal status.

Jesus' Travels as a Young Man

To initiate his trip as a young man of thirteen (after his "presentation at the temple" and "those questionings . . . of the leaders"), there was a short journey south into Egypt before his trip to India and Persia:

> [T]he entity was sent first . . . into Egypt for only a short period, and then into India, and then into what is now Persia.
> Hence in all the ways of the teachers the entity was trained.
> 5749-7

In India Jesus learned "those cleansings of the body as related to preparation for strength in the physical, as well as in the mental man." (5749-2)

(Q) From what period and how long did He remain in India?
(A) From thirteen to sixteen. One year in travel and in Persia; the greater portion being in the Egyptian.   5749-2

(Q) Please describe Jesus' education in India, schools attended—did He attend the Essene school in Jagannath taught by Lamaas, and did He study in Benares also under the Hindu teacher Udraka?
(A) He was there at least three years. Arcahia was the teacher.
                                                    2067-7

In Persia and in his travels, he studied "the unison of forces as related to those teachings . . . of Zu and Ra." (5749-2) However, a message from home, informing him of his father's death, cut short his studies there: "From Persia he was called to Judea at the death of Joseph . . . " (5749-7)
Jesus then returned to Egypt

for the completion of the preparation as teacher.
He was with John, the messenger, during the portion of the training there in Egypt.   5749-7

In Egypt, [he learned] that which had been the basis of all the teachings in those of the temple, and the after actions of the crucifying of self in relationships to ideals that made for the abilities of carrying on that called to be done.
(Q) Are there any written records which have not been found of the teachings?
(A) More, rather, of those of the close associates, and those records that are yet to be found of the preparation of the man, of the Christ, in those of the tomb, or those yet to be uncovered in the pyramid.   5749-2

(Q) Please describe Jesus' education in Egypt in Essene schools of Alexandria and Heliopolis, naming some of His outstanding teachers and subjects studied.

(A) Not in Alexandria—rather in Heliopolis, for the period of attaining to the priesthood, or the taking of the examinations there—as did John. One was in one class, one in the other.

(Q) Name some of His outstanding teachers and subjects studied.

(A) Not as teachers, but as being *examined* by these; passing the tests there. These, as they have been since their establishing, were tests through which ones attained to that place of being accepted or rejected by the influences of the mystics as well as of the various groups or schools in other lands. For, as indicated oft through this channel, the unifying of the teachings of many lands was brought together in Egypt; for that was the center from which there was to be the radial activity of influence in the earth—as indicated by the first establishing of those tests, or the recording of time as it has been, was and is to be—until the new cycle is begun.   2067-7

(Q) Tell about Judy teaching Jesus, where and what subjects she taught him, and what subjects she planned to have him study abroad.

(A) The prophecies! Where? In her home. When? During those periods from his twelfth to his fifteenth-sixteenth year, when he went to Persia and then to India. In Persia, when his father died. In India when John [the Baptist] first went to Egypt—where Jesus joined him and both became the initiates in the pyramid or temple there.

(Q) What subjects did Judy plan to have him study abroad?

(A) What you would today call astrology.   2067-11

Following Jesus' training in Egypt, he returned, then, to his home—
land . . .

to Capernaum, Cana, and those periods of the first preparation in the land of the nativity.

The rest ye have according to Mark, John, Matthew and Luke;

these in their order record most of the material experiences of
the Master.   5749-7

The picture from the readings this ultimately paints of Jesus is one of
a man who spent most of his life outside of Palestine rather than as a
resident citizen. If we count his five-year sojourn in Egypt, beginning in
his infancy (including travel time), Jesus would have spent only fifteen
years (twelve as a child and three as an adult) living within Palestine
and eighteen years as a traveling student or master in training in an
expatriate capacity (five as an infant and thirteen total as an adult). The
readings' outlook drastically overhauls the traditional view of him as a
simple laborer. Instead, he was someone who understood other cultures and traditions, who spoke numerous languages, and who passed
the tests of teachers in other religious communities to prove his exceptional spiritual capacity. He was not merely a Jew for the Jews but a
grand mystic for the world. Today his true greatness is not as a historical religious figure, as his historical relics are virtually nonexistent, but
as a transcultural mystical influence—a spiritual force whom the great
mystics of many traditions love and honor.

Just as Egypt plays an important role in the development of Judaism,
Egypt will be central to Jesus' biography. Egypt was historically an important location for his training because, if you recall the previously
noted reading, "the unifying of the teachings of many lands was brought
together in Egypt; for that was the center from which there was to be
the radial activity of influence in the earth." (2067-7)

This reframing of Jesus' biography is one of the valuable contributions the readings make to our understanding of the Christ event. It
informs our perspective with a greater scope and augments our appreciation for the greatness of this soul.

A few other notable bits are revealed in the readings relative to the
Christ event. First, the readings present the three Magi as originating
from the three countries that Jesus would later visit: Egypt, Persia, and
India. The readings' source also states that they were metaphysical em-
blems of body (gold), mind (frankincense), and soul (myrrh, or the "healing force" of myrrh), respectively. (5749-7) Also, as mentioned earlier,

there were numerous visits from many Magi, even from Babylonia and China:

> There was more than one visit of the Wise Men. [The account
> commonly known] is a record of three Wise Men. There was the
> fourth, as well as the fifth, and then the second group. They
> came from Persia, India, Egypt, and also from Chaldea, Gobi,
> and what is *now* the Indo or Tao land.   2067-7

Second, the readings state emphatically that Jesus was immaculately conceived, as was his mother, Mary.

Mary was sixteen and Joseph thirty-six at the time of their marriage. Joseph, it seems, wanted nothing to do with taking a bride so young but was convinced through dreams and metaphysical visions—both his and others'. Not until ten years after the birth of Jesus, when Mary was approximately twenty-six, did they "take up the normal life of a married couple," conceiving their next three children naturally: James, Ruth, and Jude. Jesus would have been studying in Egypt, Persia, and India at the time of his siblings' births. The readings' information is unclear as to whether Jesus traveled back to Palestine at any time during his Egyptian studies. Perhaps it was unnecessary. Judy, we are told, could project herself to distant locations. We may surmise that Jesus had already gained that skill. If this was the case, as it has been with many swamis and lamas, then communication would have been very efficient, and arduous return treks unnecessary.

Jesus, Mary, and the Close Associates

A few intriguing pieces of information emerge in the readings regarding the people who surrounded Jesus during his Palestinian mission. The readings clarify the position of the disciples as being rather well-off, certainly not destitute or poor, as the traditional myth has implied.

One reading states that Zebedee and his wife Mary, parents of John and James, were

> . . . not of the rabble, not of the political, not of great *spiritual*
> influence or force among the [community]. While both were of

the Jewish faith, as would be termed today, or the Hebraic faith, they were in that position socially which was above that of the ordinary individuals.   540-4

This reading explains that their lineages originated from the houses of Judah and Levi (although it does not state who belonged to what lineage) and that through Zebedee, the family had connections with the Essenes and those groups that "held rather to a more universality of application of the tenets and teachings of the peoples during the period." The principal idea conveyed here is that these Essenes, Jesus' Essenes, saw past their own cultural limitations and embraced sacred teachings from many areas.

The distinguished Gospel patriarch Zebedee, we are told, "was . . . in the fishing business as a wholesaler, than being in active service himself." The whole family would become involved with the Essenes after first becoming familiar with John the Baptist's teachings, then later with Jesus:

Hence not only the brothers but those employed by the brothers (Peter, Andrew and Judas—not Iscariot) joined in the [Essene] activities. These were of the fisherfolk who aided in establishing the teachings in and among the people, that held to *both* the old [Jewish customs] and the new environs [Essene universalism.]   540-4

For Zebedee first was a follower of John, then of those that had separated themselves from the Jewish Sanhedrin, the Jewish law, and of the head of the *Essenes* in those studies to which *both* John the Baptist and the Master came first as teachers, and as instructors.   1089-3

[T]he sons of Zebedee were among those sufficiently able financially, as would be termed in the present, to leave their work, their home (and all of the Apostles, save Matthew); for these, the sons of Zebedee, were in favor with those in political authority.   2946-3

> Mary the mother of Christ became a dweller in the house or home of John [the beloved, son of Zebedee]—who joined with those in Bethany; for John, as may be well known, was the wealthiest of the disciples of the Christ. His estate would be counted in the present, in American money, as being near to a quarter of a million dollars;[36] or to the estate where he was a power with those in the Roman and Jewish power at the period.
>
> 295-8

Reading 5749-15 presents some details of the wedding at Cana. It was on the third of June and for the marriage of Roael (Zebedee's son and an elder sibling to James and John) and Mary, a distant relative of Jesus' mother. The well-known incident of running out of wine was particularly acute for Jesus' mother, for she was helping host the event, and "remember, the sons of Zebedee were among those of the upper class, as would be termed; not the poorer ones."

The readings state that mother Mary needed some proof that Jesus was manifesting his spiritual connection; she was having some doubts and needed to be reassured, especially since she had been divinely guided to his care by the angels while he was still in utero:

> This might be called a first period of test. For, had He not just ten days ago sent Satan away, and received ministry from the angels? This had come to be known as hearsay. Hence the natural questioning [by] the mother-love [of His divine] purposes; this son—strange in many ways had chosen, by the dwelling in the wilderness for the forty days, and then the returning to the lowly people, the fishermen, about this country. It brought on the questioning by the mother.   5749-15

There was also quite an age range between the disciples, something that is not clarified in the traditional Gospel accounts: "Peter would be about sixty, while John would only be about eighteen, and the Master thirty-two." (3054-4)

We do not have any historical data to validate this claim in the readings, but it is included here as interesting food for thought.

Mary Magdalene

In the Gospel's summary of Jesus' three-year mission in Palestine, Mary Magdalene often goes unnamed in accounts of her actions. The readings are not definitive, as they present two women who were accused of adultery and sentenced to stoning, but it seems quite logical that the Gospel writers were repeatedly returning to Mary's story. The readings state that Mary and Martha were critical resources for historical information and Jesus' sayings.

It is clear, however, that Mary of Magdala (or Magdalene), sister of Martha and Lazarus, was a wanton woman—one who gave her body in exchange for possessions and social prestige among wealthy patrons. She was essentially the ancient equivalent of a high-class call girl:

> Mary of Magdalene . . . the courtesan that was active in the experiences both of those that were in the capacity of the Roman officers, Roman peoples, and those that were of the native lands and country . . .
>
> As to the experiences before meeting the Master, these were more of the worldly nature; wherein there was the giving of self in body, in the [indulgences] of the period, such that there was brought for the body and those associated with same the activities that brought condemnation, as well as the pomp, the power, the splendor, when considered from that angle . . .
>
> With the death and separation of the Master from the disciples (as it may be called), the home of Mary and Martha became—for the time—rather the center from which most of the activities of the disciples took place, who were of that activity; that is, who were not altogether Galileans, see?   295-8

Mary was twenty-three when "Christ cleansed her of the seven devils." This proved a turning point in her biography.

[A]nd with the return of Mary after [her spiritual] conversion and the casting out of the demons—this brought even greater confusion to the entity [993]. For, to the entity, how *could* anyone who had been *such* a person—or who had so disregarded persons [for the sake of] material gain—become an honored one among those, or in association with a household of ones such as [the esteemed] Lazarus and Martha.   993-5

Mary becomes the principal female disciple, much to the consternation of Peter, as we read in the Nag Hammadhi Gnostic gospels. This was at a time when females and males were discouraged from associating publicly, and certainly women were not to be taught with men, alongside men as equals. Jesus, while teaching Mary and energetically transforming her from a whore to a spiritual devotee, never stooped to sexual interactions.

(Q) Is it true that Jesus in His youth loved Mary, Martha's sister as a sweetheart, or did He never have a sweetheart?
(A) Mary, the sister of Martha, was an harlot—until the cleansing; and not one that Jesus would have loved, though He loved all.   2067-7

So, from the readings' view, that is the definitive answer—Jesus did not have sexual relations with Mary.

Mary was the pariah of the family and only became accepted after her "cleansing" and psychic metamorphosis. This was another validation of the transformative power of Christ Consciousness transference.

. . . as to when and how Mary had been cleansed from those activities and experiences, little of which until then had even been spoken of . . . Also the entity [2390] heard much of Martha, the one sedate, calm, never even venturing to offer her body *ever* in those activities that had made Mary the byword of so many . . .   2390-3

Mary's sister, Martha, is often presented as being uncorrupt and virtuous but still spiritually negligent for attending to household duties instead of learning from the Master. Jesus tells her that His teachings will stay with her, implying a soul-level effect. This is a common assertion by the yogic masters as well, not to allow worldly duties and enticements to pull one from God's presence or the eternal value of the spiritual path. What remains with us after physical death is not social achievement and material gain but our attunement to Spirit.

The sisters' brother, Lazarus, dies of typhoid fever—from which Jesus resurrects him. (993-5) This is an example of the yogic art of resurrection, whereby the masters sometimes pull someone back from what appears to be inescapable death. It helps teach us just how thin the line is between life and death and how much power the spirit has over the physical costume.

Jesus is directly responsible for mending the breach in the family caused by Mary's sordid behavior. People are also astounded that Jesus picks Mary, of all women, to become a disciple. His choice has validity on many levels. First, Mary had passion that was misdirected. It is easier to redirect energy than to try to procure it from nothing. Although Martha was well-behaved and socially respectable, she adhered to social convention too much to break free and, for example, publicly anoint Jesus' feet with expensive oil, as did her sister. This exemplified the degree of passion a disciple must have in order to attain deeper levels of the spiritual heart.

Second, since God forgives our numerous rebellious acts and provides with each incarnation incalculable opportunities for reconciliation, Jesus was modeling this Divine benevolence for all to behold. Mary was an ideal beneficiary because she had both ardor and culpability and could, with the impetus of her passion, redirect her consciousness toward God, thus nullifying her mistakes.

Third, Jesus was influenced by women and knew that holiness and enlightenment were not biased toward gender. He saw past the physical costume and wanted others to do the same. Turning a harlot into a spiritual devotee embodies the incomprehensible power of God consciousness, showing that in God's eyes, every single soul is equally precious and capable of at-one-ment with God.

Jesus: The Man, His Mission

The historical Jesus was an enlightened being, a mystic with a cosmopolitan view of spiritual truths and yet very down to earth:

> He wined, He dined with the rich; He consorted with the poor, He entered the temple on state occasions, yea He slept in the field with the shepherds, yea He walked by the seashore with the throngs, He preached to those in the mount—*all things*; and yet ever ready to present the tenets, the truths, even in those forms of tales . . . parables . . . activities that took hold upon the *lives of men and women* in *every* walk of human experience!   1472-3

The Humorous Side of Jesus

> Merry—even in the hour of trial. Joke—even in the moment of betrayal.   5749-1

> Cultivate the ability to see the ridiculous, and to retain the ability to laugh. For, know—only in those that God hath favored is there the ability to laugh, even when clouds of doubt arise, or when every form of disturbance arises. For, remember, the Master smiled—and laughed, oft—even on the way to Gethsemane.
>
>   2984-1

One unique contribution the readings offer is a view of the light-hearted side of Jesus. As with all great masters, they employ humor liberally, and Jesus was no exception. The view that we accept of him today—the suffering, betrayals, and losses—was principally shaped during medieval times. One device that the Jewish tradition employs wonderfully is a fanciful and clever use of humor as a teaching tool. This goes back to some of the oldest Jewish texts. Jesus would have been very familiar with this tradition and amply used humor to both teach and amuse.

Such humor is commonly found in Hebrew and Arabic writings as puns and other wordplay. The marvelous translations of the Gospels by George Lamsa shed light on this, as he explains the numerous puns present in the Aramaic (Jesus' native tongue) versions of the Gospel narratives. As Buddhist lamas and Indian yogis have personified for centuries, the closer in consciousness one gets to God, the more this world appears as a play or a Divine farce. This world, we are told by those who know, is just God's shtick—don't be a schlemiel, but don't take it too seriously either. This would be at par with Jesus' mindset—the one we see in the readings.

One True of Purpose

> Even in Elijah or John we find the faltering, the doubting. We find no faltering, no doubting, no putting aside of the purpose in the Master Jesus.   3054-4

Consistently, in the readings, the crystal-clear picture is painted of Jesus unwavering in his spiritual purpose: To rectify all outstanding personal karma, absorb and transform mass karma, and be a shining example of how to achieve enlightenment. His studies and influences from other cultures helped him achieve this aim. This great yogi saw past material trappings, the illusion of physical limitations, and institutional dogma. While being very human, his consciousness was perfectly attuned to God.

His spirituality was simple and pragmatic, cutting to the heart of what was necessary for enlightenment:

> He set no rules of appetite. He set no rules of ethics, other than, "As ye would that men should do to you, do ye so even to them," and to know "Inasmuch as ye do it unto the least of these, thy brethren, ye do it unto thy Maker." He declared that the kingdom of heaven is within each entity's consciousness, to

be attained, to be aware of—through meditating upon the fact
that God is the Father of every soul.   357-13

Just as the great swamis teach, something created you—what or who
is it? You have not come out of nothing—from where have you come?
We must dive deeply within ourselves to uncover these answers, as
they exist within our consciousness. This is what spiritual yoga, the
yoga of the Christ, facilitates.

18

The Reincarnated Christ

Jesus, in his previous incarnations, plays critical roles in the formation of Judeo–Christian thought. The soul we now call Jesus was unquestionably central, in his previous lives, to the development of Jewish theology. The readings state that he, as a reincarnating soul, was responsible for the lion's share of Jewish history and mythology in the Tanakh (the Holy Scriptures of Judaism).

But when or if the entity takes this as its study (and set this as its thought and then read, then study the Book which tells of Him, Jesus born in Bethlehem of the Virgin Mary), know this is the same soul-entity who reasoned with those who returned from captivity in those days when Nehemiah, Ezra, Zerubbabel were factors in the attempts of the reestablishing of the worship of God [in the rebuilt Jerusalem temple], [known in that incarnation as] **Jeshua**, the scribe, [who] translated the rest of the books written up to that time. Then realize that is the same entity . . . who as **Joshua** was the mouthpiece [. . . Exodus 12-18] of Moses, who gave the law, and was the same soul-entity who was born in Bethlehem, the same soul-entity who in those periods of the strength and yet the weakness of Jacob in his love for Rachael was their firstborn **Joseph**. This is the same

entity . . . who had manifested to father Abraham as the prince, as the priest of Salem, without father and without mother, without days or years [**Melchizedek**, Genesis 14:18], but a living human being in flesh made manifest in the earth from the desire of Father-God to prepare an escape for man [I Cor. 10:13], as was warned by the same entity as **Enoch**, and this was also the entity **Adam**. And this was the spirit of light.   5023-2
[last three bracketed comments original to reading; boldface, author's]

Ye have seen it in Adam; ye have heard it in Enoch, ye have had it made known in Melchizedek; Joshua, Joseph . . . and those that made the preparation then for him called Jesus. [. . . See Malachi 3 and 4] Ye have seen His Spirit in the leaders in all realms of activity, whether in the isles of the sea, the wilderness, the mountain, or in the various activities of every race, every color, every activity of that which has produced and does produce contention in the minds and hearts of those that dwell in the flesh.   5749-5 [brackets in original]

The story of this entire cycle, Jesus as the first "Adam" to the last messiach, is a multifaceted one in the readings and not without its inherent enigmas. Still, it helps explain why some of the Gnostic Christians referred to Jesus as the "last Adam," as being "in the spirit of Melchizedek," and as one "imbued with the power of Enoch."

For know that He . . . [the same one] who was lifted up on the Cross in Calvary—was also . . . he that first walked among men at the beginning of man's advent into flesh! For He indeed was and is the first Adam, the last Adam; that is the way, the truth, the light!   2402-2

Culling through the readings, we have to piece together the fragmentary data of the Christ event like a jigsaw puzzle. Essentially, the story goes something like this:

Once upon a time, when God's creations (we humans, but still in spirit form) were given the use of free will by the Godhead, something peculiar happened. The creations decided to exercise their free will to move away from the Godhead and explore their own individuality, their own power to create. This resulted in the creation of a mind. Spirit projected into an individualized, self-contained unit in what we now call "mind."

These spirits-with-mind eventually projected themselves into the earth plane. A significant inspiration for doing so seemed to be this powerful entity named Amelius (eventually to have a life as Jesus.) Thousands of years passed, and the spirits-with-mind created numerous problems projecting themselves into matter. It seems that plenty of glitches appeared—the spirits were being trapped in matter, no longer able to come and go as they once could. There was also the problem of their getting addicted to the enjoyment of their carnal experiences and the use of their free will. The entire system had to eventually be redesigned, with Amelius as architect. A new physical body was then created and was now "Adam," which in Hebrew (*adamah*) means "clay," or "earth." This would be a body with a specific birth and death experience, what we now experience as an incarnation.

The *adamah* eventually gets split into two, and what is commonly called "Eve"—*hawwah* in Hebrew, meaning "life-bearer"—is created. The word commonly (mis)translated as "rib" also means "side," so actually, the story goes, "Clay-earth had a side of it turned into life-bearer." The words *adam* and *eve* were not given names but mythological concepts. The readings state that the process of creating male and female humans from a unified spiritual form took eighty-six years. (364-7)

So the new incarnations were "adamah," or "clay"—masses of protein and water—containers for spirit. The addiction and obsession with these bodies held the individual spirits in exile from the Godhead and eventually had to be deconstructed by the one who instigated its design, the soul that we now know as Jesus.

> [T]hough He were the first of man, the first of the sons of God in spirit, in flesh, it became necessary that He fulfill *all* those associations, those [karmic] connections that were to wipe away in

> the experience of man that which separates him from his Maker.
>   5749-6

> Thus is He the only begotten, the firstborn, the first to know
> flesh, the first to purify it.   1158-5

The eventual destruction of his body on a cross would be a symbolic ending to his role as the first *adamah*. Once this somatic termination occurred, all other earthbound spirits could follow his lead by choosing a spiritual consciousness over a material one. This is the path enthusiastically endorsed by the readings' source—the sacrificial path of Christ Consciousness.

Christ Consciousness is the forgetting of self's needs and desires in complete surrender to love . . .

> [that] universal consciousness of love that we see manifested in
> those who have forgotten self . . . [and] give themselves that
> others may know the truth.   1376-1

This spiritual state is the result of attuning our conscious mind with the subconscious and, eventually, superconscious mind in deep meditative states:

> [Illumination, or Christ Consciousness] is found . . . by the open-
> ing of those channels within the physical body through which
> the energies of the Infinite are attuned to the centers through
> which physical consciousness, mental activity, is attained—or
> in deep meditation.   2109-2

This also helps clarify why the readings state that there were five "Adams" simultaneously. Since *adamah* is referring to the new incarnating bodies, the five races could have developed simultaneously, which the readings affirm they did.

Jesus as the Mythical Enoch:
"And God Took Him Home"

Enoch has a brief appearance in the Tanakh, but his influence would be felt for subsequent centuries. In Genesis 5:18–24 all we get is this:

> When Jared was 162 years old, Enoch was born. Jared lived after the birth of Enoch 800 years, and had other sons and daughters . . . When Enoch was 65 years old, Methuselah was born. Enoch walked [in habitual fellowship] with God after the birth of Methuselah 300 years and had other sons and daughters. So all the days of Enoch were 365 years. And Enoch walked [in habitual fellowship] with God; and he was not, for God took him [home with Him.]

The name Enoch is commonly translated from Hebrew as "dedicated," or "consecrated," and comes from the Hebrew root *chanak*, meaning "to initiate discipline." We could also say that Enoch means "initiator," as in a priest who initiates or consecrates disciples.

As Enoch, he (the soul–entity Jesus) first overcomes death (Hebrews 11:5) and sets the stage for a significant part of early Jewish mysticism. Enoch, the great–grandfather of Noah, is presented as having lived 365 years. (Genesis 5) The correspondence to the number of days in the solar year cannot be overlooked. *The Books of Enoch* are known by many biblical scholars to have been highly influential in early Judeo–Christian spirituality:

> Enochian authority Dr. R.H. Charles noted some years ago that "the influence of Enoch on the New Testament has been greater than that of all the other apocryphal and pseudepigraphical books taken together." *The Ethiopian Book of Enoch* is considered to have been Paul's constant reference book; John was quite affected by Enoch, especially in Revelation; and Peter's letters in the New Testament reflect the considerable influence of Enoch.[37]

Enoch was a mystic of high caliber and a scribe. What exactly he recorded is unknown, but it seems that many parts of the mystical theology found in the Torah can be traced, directly or indirectly, to the influence of Enoch.[38]

The earliest extracanonical or pseudigraphical work attributed to Enoch is found in the *Ethiopian Book of Enoch*, also called *The Book of I Enoch*. It is an amalgamated document consisting of teachings scholars believe to have been written between the third century BCE and the first century CE. According to biblical scholars, "The only complete copy was found in an Ethiopic translation in the eighteenth century" and is known to once have been widely regarded by Jews and Christians alike. "Aramaic fragments of the book have been found among the Dead Sea Scrolls and at Masada, the Herodian fortress where the last survivors of the Jewish Revolt against Rome perished about 73 C.E. Apparently accepted in some Christian circles of antiquity, I Enoch is quoted as Scripture in the New Testament epistle of Jude."[39] The Book of Enoch foreshadows apocalyptic ideas that emerge later in Daniel, Isaiah, and the Revelation of John. I Enoch also creates the connection between Adam (portrayed by a white bull) and the Messiah (the lamb). The bull is symbolic of fertility and virility and, in this context, the creation of bodies for karmic reconciliation. The lamb is symbolic of sacrifice, of surrendering the physical experience to return home in God consciousness.

Enoch is employed as a mystical archetype by early Judeo–Christian teachers. Writing in his name was not uncommon as a means of conveying the spirit of Enochian wisdom or metaphysical theology/cosmology. He is emblematic of one who does not need to physically die in order to return to a heavenly state.

> How does prayer reach the throne of mercy or grace, or that from which it emanates? From itself! Through that of *crucifying*, *nullifying*, the carnal mind and opening the mental in such a manner that the Spirit of truth may flow in its psychic sense, or occult force, into the very being, that you may be one with that from which you came! Be thou faithful unto that committed into

thy keeping! Life *itself* is precious! For why? It is of the Maker itself! That *is* the beginning! The psychic forces, the attunements, the developments, going *to* that! As did many in that experience. And Enoch walked with God, and he was not for God took him. As [were] many of those in those first years, in this land, this experience.   364-10

In reading 1158-5, the Cayce source specifies that three people have come to earth and "entered into flesh *without* that act which man knows as copulation": Enoch, Melchizedek, and Jesus.

First find thyself. Apply thyself in such a way and manner as to know what ye will do with this man, Jesus of Nazareth—Jeshua of Jerusalem, Joshua in Shiloh, Joseph in the court of Pharaoh, Melchizedek, as he blessed Abraham, Enoch as he warned the people, Adam as he listened to Eve.
3054-4

Again it [the spiritual ideal of God consciousness] was manifested in Enoch, who oft sought to walk and talk with that divine influence; with the abilities latent and manifested in self to find self in the varied realms of awareness, yet using the office of relationships as a channel through which blessings might come, as well as recommendations and warnings might be indicated to others.   2072-4

In other words, Enoch was a kind of Semitic shaman, as we might conceive of it today.

Enoch was a teacher of universal spiritual laws—means by which incarnated humans could find a way to spiritual freedom. The readings' source recommended to some people that they study "the law proclaimed by Enoch (found mostly in Jude and in the early chapters of Genesis)." (3653-1)

Jesus as the Mystical Priest Melchizedek

As the priestly king, Melchizedek establishes the payment of tithes and the symbolic use of bread and wine, continued today as the Eucharist. It appears that Melchizedek was either a spontaneous manifestation or a mystic unconcerned with lineage:

> He is primarily, as his name when translated indicates, king of righteousness, and then he is also king of Salem, which means king of peace. Without [record of] father or mother or ancestral line, neither with beginning days nor ending of life, but, resembling the Son of God, he continues to be a priest without interruption and without successor.   Hebrews 7:2-3

In Hebrew his name would mean either "king of righteousness" or perhaps "righteous king." Some scholars also believe that a connection can be made between the Canaanite deity Zedek and the name Melchizedek, which could mean "my king is Zedek." Zedek is also the Hebrew name for Jupiter, adding an interesting astrological component to his legacy. Traditionally, Melchizedek is thought of as a mystical priest of ancient Jerusalem.

Historical records validate that Jerusalem used to be known as Uru-Salem [shalom] or just Salem.

> You are a priest for ever [according to] the manner and order of Melchizedek.   Psalm 110:4

> Hence the group we refer to here as the Essenes, which was the outgrowth of the periods of preparations from the teachings by Melchizedek, as propagated by Elijah and [Elisha] and Samuel. These were set aside for preserving themselves in direct line of choice for the offering of themselves as channels through which there might come the new or the divine origin, see?   254-109

The following passage in Hebrews suggests knowledge of Melchizedek as a former incarnation of Jesus:

> Where Jesus has entered in for us [in advance], a Forerunner
> having become a High Priest forever after the order of
> Melchizedek.
>   Hebrews 6:20

Knowing that Melchizedek was both a priest and a king gives special poignancy to Jesus being crucified as the "King of the Jews." Certainly, for those who mocked the notion of reincarnation, this would have been a cruel enjoyment to see the supposed reincarnated Melchizedek, the great mystical priest, dying as a common criminal. And this would have been more disdainful fuel for the fire against Jesus, since he or his followers claimed he was once Melchizedek, a larger-than-life figure in Jewish mythology.

The Abraham–Melchizedek connection is important in the Letter to the Hebrews:

> For this Melchizedek, king of Salem [and] priest of the Most
> High God, met Abraham as he returned from the slaughter of
> the kings and blessed him. And Abraham gave to him a tenth
> portion of all [the spoil] . . . Now observe and consider how
> great [a personage] this was to whom even Abraham the patri-
> arch gave a tenth—the topmost [the pick] of the heap—of the
> spoils.
>   Hebrews 7:1-2, 4

Contrast this with the reported words of Jesus:

> I assure you, most solemnly I tell you, if any one observes My
> teaching . . . he will by no means ever see and experience death.
>   The Jews said to Him, Now we know that You are under the
> power of a demon [insane]. Abraham died and also the proph-
> ets; yet You say, If a man keeps My word he will never taste of
> death to all eternity.
>   Are You greater than our father Abraham? He died and all the
> prophets died! Who do You make Yourself out to be?
>   Jesus answered, If I were to glorify Myself, I should have no
> real glory . . . It is My Father Who glorifies Me . . . of Whom you

say that He is your God.

Yet you do not know Him nor recognize Him . . .

Your forefather Abraham was extremely happy at the hope and prospect of seeing My day [My incarnation] . . . And he did see it and was delighted.

Then the Jews said to Him, You are not yet fifty years old, and have You seen Abraham?

Jesus replied, I assure you, I most solemnly tell you, before Abraham was born, I AM.   John 8:51-58

The Gnostic tract *Melchizedek*, discovered in the Nag Hammadhi find of 1945, reflects the commonly held belief in Egyptian Gnosticism that Melchizedek and Jesus were one and the same soul. This is sometimes referred to as a product of Sethian Gnosticsm, but the truth is that numerous Gnostic sects understood this connection. The *Melchizedek* tract is very fragmented, with only 19 lines of text intact out of some 745. Still, it is clear, upon studying this Gnostic text, that the author(s) were undeniably making the connection between Christ and Melchizedek:

You crucified me from the third hour on the Sabbath eve until the ninth hour. And after these things I arose from the dead . . . They said to me, "Be strong, O Melchizedek, great High-priest of God, Most High . . . who are your enemies [that] have made war, you have prevailed over them and they did not prevail over you and you endured . . . " [40]

It seems that as Adam (*adamah*), Enoch, and Melchizedek, the soul-entity Jesus was laying the spiritual foundations of what was to come later in his final incarnation. The following Cayce reading hints that both Enoch and Melchizedek were kinds of archetypes:

First, in the beginning, of course; and then as Enoch, Melchizedek, in the perfection. Then in the earth of Joseph, Joshua, Jeshua, Jesus.   5749-14

> Again there may be drawn to self a parallel from the realm of spiritual enlightenment of that entity known as Melchizedek, a prince of peace, one seeking ever to be able to bless those in their judgments who have sought to become channels for a helpful influence without any seeking for material gain, or mental or material glory; but magnifying the virtues, minimizing the faults in the experiences of all with whom the entity comes in contact day by day.   2072-4

It appears that as both Enoch and Melchizedek, he was able to dematerialize at will; neither figures are known to have died a natural human death.

> First, He was created—brought into being from all that there was in the earth, as an encasement for the soul of an entity, a part of the Creator; knowing separation in death. Then He was [born] through the union of channels growing out of that thought of the Creator made manifest . . . as Enoch as to merit the escaping of death—which had been the result as the law of disobedience. He was made manifest in Melchizedek by desire alone, not knowing body, not knowing mind—save its own; brought into being in materialization as of itself; passing from materialization in the same manner.   2072-4

Biblical scholars realize the connection Melchizedek has to the Essenes via the Dead Sea Scrolls. In a notable section called by many "The War Scrolls," the totality of humanity is separated into two basic factions—"the children of righteousness and light" and "the children of falsehood and darkness." In the midst of a cosmic battle between the two, Melchizedek "will destroy Satan and all his minions and judge all those, human and angels, who served evil and defied the good."[41] This is reminiscent of Jesus' use of light–versus–darkness metaphors in the Gospels:

> You are the light of the world . . . Let your light so shine before

men . . . that they may praise and glorify your Father who is in
heaven.   Matthew 5:14,16

[T]he Light has come into the world, and people have loved the
darkness rather than . . . the Light.   John 3:19

Walk while you have the Light . . . so that darkness may not
overtake you. He who walks about in the dark does not know
where he goes. While you have the Light, believe in the Light
. . . that you may become [children] of the Light.
                                                         John 12:35-36

According to the readings, there are two significant contributions
that Melchizedek makes: Writing the Book of Job and establishing the
spiritual tenets that the Essenes will later employ.

Jesus as Joseph, Son of Jacob:
The Paragon of Forgiveness

In Hebrew, Yosef (Joseph) means "God will give the increase" or, in
some versions, "It is up to the Lord to supplement."

Joseph plays an important role as a man of great moral strength and
spiritual integrity and is a paragon of forgiveness. There are some remarkable parallels between his incarnation as Joseph and as Jesus. Both
men had to flee to Egypt as an important means of self-preservation
and, ultimately, transformation. Cayce reports that the Jesus soul had
numerous Egyptian connections—finding refuge in Egypt as an infant,
and his discipleship and empowerment as a young man, in preparation
for his Palestinian mission.

Both Jesus and Joseph forgave their close allies for their aggression
and violence. Just as Jesus started his Palestinian scenario at age thirty,
Joseph will begin his service to the king at age thirty. (Sanderfur, 98)

Jesus as Joshua, Moses' Military Aide:
One Who Lived by the Sword

For Joshua was the interpreter through whom the message was
given to Israel.   3645-1

. . . the patient Joshua, the one who followed closely in the way
that would give to the individual (who would study) the life and
interpretation of the Son of man. These in the earth activity
were much alike (Joshua and Jesus) not as combative, as in the
warrings, but in spirit and in purpose, in ideals, these were one.
                                                              3409-1

. . . Joshua the prophet, the mystic, the leader, the incarnation
of the Prince of Peace.   362-1

Joshua begins his life with the name Hosea ("salvation"), but Moses
changes it to Joshua (Yeshua in Hebrew: "God saves" or "God's salvation"), reminiscent of how Jesus will change Peter's name, spurring his
discipleship. This was an extremely popular name during the Jewish
return from Babylonian exile, the Second Temple era. It is a contracted
form of Yehoshua, which, if taken literally, can translate to "God help us
now!"

In Matthew 1:21, "the angel of the Lord" instructs Mary this way:
"[Y]ou shall call his name Jesus [in Hebrew means Savior], for He will
save His people from their sins." Joshua will both save the Israelites
(from the Canaanites) and the writings of the Torah. Jeshua will save
both the temple and the post-exile mythology. Jesus will save the spirits
trapped in matter by creating an end to the ancient cycle of karmic
rebirths.

As Joshua, his incarnation is filled with stories of righteous battles.
The first time that the concept of a biblical "holy war" appears is with
Joshua. From the author's perspective, YHWH (God) is prepared to destroy any of Israel's enemies as long as the Israelites remain faithful to
the Mosaic covenant, which entails the people staying faithful to the

mitzvot, or divine commandments of YHWH. Joshua is recorded as insti-
gating thirty-one military campaigns.

At the beginning of Joshua's military career, it was a harlot named
Rahab that gave Joshua's two spies cover against the king of Jericho.
(Joshua 2:1) This act would spare her and her family when Joshua and
his army returned to burn the city and steal all the gold, silver, brass
and iron, which they had "put into the treasury of the house of the
Lord." (Joshua 6:24) Some sources state that Joshua married Rahab, but
that is not explicit in the Book of Joshua.

This episode, and the following one, would foreshadow an important
act of repentance and forgiveness with Jesus, incarnated as Joshua. A
man named Achan had stolen from Joshua and the people. This caused
the Joshuan army to lose an important battle at the village of Ai. As
punishment, the man was first burned alive and then stoned by Joshua's
troops. When Mary Magdelene was brought before Jesus to be stoned
for her adultery, he encouraged forgiveness instead of retribution. All
throughout his incarnation as Jesus, he is rectifying his karmic debts of
the past. The readings state that there were two such episodes of forgiveness—one with Mary and another with a woman accused of associating with a Roman soldier. Interestingly, in the reading that mentions
the second case of adultery, Jesus is said to have written in Latin.

Joshua's murder ranking is unsurpassed by anyone in the Bible (not
counting YHWH)—he was the ultimate Semitic terrorist. Some twelve
thousand men and women of Ai were slaughtered and their city burned
into "a heap of ruins for ever . . . " (Joshua 8:25,28) We do not know the
ultimate death toll, but thirty-one kings were documented as defeated,
and a population associated with each. Even though the mandate "Thou
shalt not kill" is part of the Mosaic covenant, Joshua is justified because
he is following God's supposed decrees. Cayce states that Jesus is linked
with Joshua in their shared determination to do God's will, but not in
their promotion of violence. Jesus would later rectify this karma by
freely healing all around Joshua's combat region. In the life as Jesus,
this karmic debt would be paid in Jesus' healing ministrations and
teaching in many of the same areas where he previously "lived by the
sword," around and near the Sea of Galilee.

Three miraculous events are recorded in the Book of Joshua, all of which have future significance for the Christ. First, the Jordan river is cut off from the waters "coming down from above" so that the "priests bearing the ark of the covenant" can now stand "firm on dry ground in the midst of the Jordan . . . " (Joshua 3:13–17) This was for allowing the passage of the Israelites to carry the ark and for Joshua to continue his ruthless military campaigns on the Canaanites. Jesus would insist on being baptized in the Jordan River. During the baptism a "dove" descended on him, signifying a spiritual dispensation from God as redeemer. As Jesus, the baptism would be symbolic of pursuing peace and healing, countering his previous military exploits as Joshua.

The second supernatural event was the fall of Jericho's walls. It does not say how many people were killed, just that "they utterly destroyed all that was in the city, both man and woman, young and old, and ox, and sheep, and ass, with the edge of the sword." (Joshua 6) This also previews Jesus counseling Peter to put away his dagger because "all that live by the sword, die by the sword." As Jesus, he would see the folly of violence, especially if one thinks he is being directed by God, as Joshua did. Jesus tells his antagonists that he could call upon a legion of angels to assist him and defeat his foes, but he does not choose to do so—force is not the right way to reconcile conflict; his punishment from the Garden of Gethsemane to Golgotha was a painful karmic debt to validate this.

The third unusual feat was that the sun and moon were stopped for a day: "And the sun stood still, and the moon stayed, until the nation took vengeance upon their enemies." (Joshua 10:13) This would return in a new form during the crucifixion drama. From the view of the Gospels' writers, the heavens reflected the Messiach's anxiety: "It was now about the sixth hour [midday], and the darkness enveloped the whole land until the ninth hour [about three o'clock in the afternoon] . . . While the sun's light was darkened; and the curtain [of the Holy of Holies] of the temple was torn in two." (Luke 23:44–45) From the light of the star at His birth to the darkening of the sun at his murder, the mythology associated with Jesus is that the heavens and the Light of God were involved in his destiny.

There is also an interesting connection with the Cayce readings at the end of Luke. Jesus returns to the disciples after the crucifixion and says, "This is what I told you while I was still with you, that everything which is written concerning Me in the law of Moses [Torah] and the prophets [as Joshua] and the Psalms [which he largely penned as Asaph] must be fulfilled." (Luke 24:44; author's brackets) This suggests that Jesus was conveying to the disciples what the readings state about his legacy: he was a scribe or a compiler for a large part of the Tanakh.

The Cayce readings link Jesus in his past lives with each of these biblical sections: as Joshua, he will write most of the Torah and play a key role with the prophets, demanding that the Israelites be faithful to YHWH or pay the consequences. As Asaph, he will write a large portion of the Psalms, even though Asaph is actually credited only with Psalms 50 and 73–83. Psalms 77, 80, and 81 make reference to Joseph, another incarnation of Jesus. The ancient groups of liturgical devotees from King David's reign were known as the "sons of Asaph." These were likely a spiritual guild that continued on after the death of Asaph. Asaph was a mystic, scribe, and musician. Jesus played the harp at the Last Supper in accompaniment to Psalm 91, according to the Cayce readings, harkening back to his latent gifts.

We do not get clues of Joshua being a scribe in the traditional accounts. Joshua is presented as Moses' "minister," warrior and, quite likely, interpreter. The Cayce readings say that Jesus' determination to do God's will was greatly strengthened in his incarnation as Joshua. The narratives of the two incarnations, Joshua and Jesus, seem to hold important parallels, except for the fact that Joshua was a military commander with countless slain lives as part of his karmic debt.

Joshua would probably be viewed today as a religious fanatic gone terrorist. As shocking as this may seem, the stories of his bloody conquests and humiliation of his enemies validate this. The karma that would have to be paid would later manifest as the need to endure a painful and bloody humiliation at the hands of his captors, which occurred in his future lifetime as Jesus. Of course, Jesus knew that this karmic debt must be rectified, and this is why he repeatedly told his close disciples to "do what needs to be done" in spite of the difficult and painful nature of it; he will transform personal and group karma in his final incarnation.

The warrior nature of Joshua is symbolic of the willpower usurping the commands of the ego (selfishness). Amalek, the old Hebraic symbol for the devil, is the first conquest of Joshua. This is emblematic of the willpower usurping the selfish nature of the ego and obeying one's Higher Self.

> And Joshua mowed down and disabled Amalek and his people with the sword.
> And the Lord said to Moses, Write this for a memorial in the book, and rehearse it in the ears of Joshua, that I will utterly blot out the remembrance of Amalek from under the heavens . . .
> And he said, Because theirs is a hand against the throne of the Lord, the Lord will have war with Amalek from generation to generation.   Exodus 17:13-14; 16

It is the spiritual tenacity of Joshua and his complete obedience to Spirit that will serve as an important platform for his subsequent incarnation as the Christ.

According to the readings, Joshua is said to be the author of the largest part of the Torah, the first five books of the Jewish Bible. As a teacher, Jesus was not known to write anything, but in his previous lives, he served in very important scribal capacities, contributing a significant portion of the Jewish Bible.

Seen as a historical figure through modern sensibilities, Joshua is viewed as a disturbing figure—initiating the concept of a "holy war" in the Bible and ruthlessly killing and humiliating his enemies. Seen as a symbolic archetype, Joshua is the "holy fire" that triumphs over selfishness, which is our "Amalek" that keeps us distanced from God consciousness.

Jesus as Asaph:
The Artisan and Scribe of King David's Court

Another significant scribal incarnation of Jesus was as Asaph, the musician and visionary in King David's court. (See readings 364-7 and 364-8.) Asaph means "collector" or "gatherer" in Hebrew and likely reflects the fact that Asaph was the court scribe, poet, and historian.

> The Biblical Asaph became a legendary figure in both Jewish and Muslim literature. He is presented as master of occult arts, a princely figure, a medical master, the confidant of King Solomon, and one who knew the Ineffable Name of God, one who had the power to perform miracles.[42]

A dozen of the 150 Psalms are attributed to Asaph's creation. It is likely that he wrote many more as one presenting in the spirit of David. This was a commonplace approach to literature and art at the time and not thought of as plagiaristic but, rather, reverential. The Cayce readings state that Jesus was a musician and played a lyre. He is presented on a few occasions singing psalms with the disciples.

Jesus as Jeshua the High Priest: The Temple Builder

The next important role in which Jesus incarnated was Jeshua, the high priest and son of Jozadek (or Jehozadek). He serves as a key chronicler of the development of the Israelites and their Jewish mythology, accounting for the time the wandering tribes establish Jerusalem through the rebuilding and rededication of the temple. This is a critical time in the Israelites' history.

Jeshua is a central figure, along with Nehemiah, Ezra, and Zerubbabel, in restoring the self-esteem and spiritual inspiration of the Jewish people after their Babylonian exile and humiliation. This same consciousness would be present in Jesus as he encouraged others to live their faith in a greater way, to dedicate themselves to God's way and to surrender their selfishness to God consciousness.

Because Jesus is reported by the Cayce source to have had three incarnations with the same name, Yeshua, we will distinguish each by calling Moses' right-hand man Joshua, the high priest during Zerubbabel's reign Jeshua, and the final messiach as Jesus.

As Jeshua, he is responsible for helping to rebuild the temple destroyed by Nebuchadnezzar's troops in 587 BCE. The Second Temple Period occurred after the return of the Jews from exile in 538 BCE by decree of Cyrus the Great, the Persian ruler of the region at that time (2 Chronicles 36:22–23). Permission to reconstruct the temple is mentioned by Haggai and Zechariah as examples of God's "favor" toward the Jews, allowing them to rebuild in spite of opposition from their neighbors.

Relative to the later incarnation as Jesus, both Joseph and Jesus are referred to as "builders," what is commonly translated as "carpenters." Jesus' metaphor for reconstructing his "temple" is a source of accusation in Matthew's Gospel account:

> At last two men came forward
> And testified, This Fellow [Jesus] said, I am able to tear down the sanctuary of the temple of God and to build it up again in three days.
> And the high priest stood up and said, Have you no answer to make? What about this that these men testify against You?
> But Jesus kept silent . . .   Matthew 26:60-63

Jesus will reinterpret the meaning of *holy temple* as the body itself. The Messiah will be emblematic of the higher self, and the "new Jerusalem" will mean a brand new state of spiritual consciousness. Interpreted from a spiritual view, this is indeed what new Jerusalem means.

Jesus as Interreligious Progenitor of Monotheism

The revelation of Jesus' past lives is an important one in the readings, as it demonstrates that he had to perfect himself in the numerous cycles of life-death reincarnations just like all humans. Many of the places in which Jesus lived in previous lives he visited during his travels as a young man. This was his time to wrap up all loose ends, completing his karmic debts in total. We are told in the readings that Jesus had the fewest possible number of incarnations: thirty. Over half of those incarnations are not given in the readings, but some interesting clues are presented that lead us to ponder, if not in mere conjecture, what role that soul played in world religious development:

(Q) What part did Jesus play in any of His reincarnations in the development of the basic teachings of the following religions and philosophies? First, Buddhism:
(A) This is just one.
(Q) Mohammedanism, Confucianism, Shintoism, Brahmanism, Platoism, Judaism.
(A) As has been indicated, the entity—as an entity—influenced either directly or indirectly all those forms of philosophy or religious thought that taught God was One . . .
     Whether in Buddhism, Mohammedanism, Confucianism, Platoism, or what—these have been added to much from that as was given by Jesus in His walk in Galilee and Judea. In all of these, then, there is that same impelling spirit. What individuals have done, do do, *to* the principles or the spirit of same—in turning this aside to meet their *own* immediate needs in material planes, or places has made for that as becomes an outstanding thing, as a moralist or the head of any independent religious force or power; for, as has been given, "Know, O Israel, the Lord thy God is *One!*" whether this is directing one of the Confucius' thought, Brahman thought, Buddha thought, Mohammedan thought; these are as teachers or representatives, or to make more of the distinct change—as was in that as given by the apostle to the gentiles: "I hear there are divisions among you. Some say I am Paul, another I am Apollos, another I am of Caiaphas. Paul may minister, Apollos may have watered, but it's *God* that gives the increase!"   364-9

(Q) In the Persian experience as San (or Zend) did Jesus give

the basic teachings of what became Zoroastrianism?
(A) In all those periods that the basic principle was the Oneness
of the Father, He has walked with men.   364-8

This consciousness of oneness, we are told in the readings, is the
ideal—this is the premier road to enlightenment, to spiritual liberation.

[F]or "my yoke is easy, my burden is light" is *seldom* understood. When the desire and the purpose [and] application [are]
one—then it becomes easy; but when they are at variance one
to another, hard *is* the way, and the call of the flesh becomes
strong.   538-30

"My yoke [yoga] is easy," the master stated. Like many yogis that followed him, his emphasis on oneness serves as an example of spiritual
yoga, reuniting (yoking) with the Source of all existence.

Notes

Chapter 1

1. George Feuerstein, *The Yoga Tradition: Its History, Literature, Philosophy and Practice* (Prescott, AZ: Bhavana Books and Prints, 1998), 287.

Chapter 2

2. In set–off, nonbiblical quotations, brackets are author's unless otherwise noted.

3. All biblical quotations are taken from The Amplified Bible unless the King James (Authorized) Version [KJV] is noted. Brackets in biblical quotations, unless otherwise specified, are original to source.

4. Paramahansa Yogananda, *God Talks with Arjuna: The Bhagavad Gita, Royal Science of God-Realization* (Los Angeles, CA: Self–Realization Fellowship, 1995), 960.

5. Ibid., 430.

6. Ibid., 961.

7. Ibid., 93.

8. Swami Nikhilananda, comp., *Vivekananda: The Yogas and Other Works* (New York, NY: Ramakrishna–Vivekananda Center, 1984), 205.

9. Yogananda, *God Talks*, 488.

10. Yogananda, *The Divine Romance* (Los Angeles, CA: Self–Realization Fellowship, 1988), 329.

Chapter 3

11. Ibid.

12. Yogananda, *God Talks*, 968.

13. Yogananda, *Divine Romance*, 311.

14. Yogananda, *God Talks*, 959.

15. Nikhilananda, *Vivekananda*, 524.

16. Yogananda, *God Talks*, 655.

17. Nikhilananda, *Vivekananda*, 214–215.

18. David Godman, ed., *Be As You Are: The Teachings of Sri Ramana Maharshi* (New York: Penguin Books, 1985), 64.

19. Nikhilananda, trans., *The Gospel of Sri Ramakrishna.* (New York, NY:

Ramakrishna–Vivekananda Center, 1984), 255.

20. Nikhilananda, *Vivekananda*, 438.

21. Yogananda, *Divine Romance*, 16–17.

Chapter 4

22. The Leydig cells, discovered in 1850 by the German anatomist Franz Leydig, are located in the testicles and are related to producing testosterone.

23. James M. Robinson, ed., *The Nag Hammadhi Library*, 3rd ed. (San Francisco, CA: Harper, 1988), 210.

Chapter 6

24. Yogananda, *Man's Eternal Quest* (Los Angeles, CA: Self–Realization Fellowship, 1988), 131.

Chapter 10

25. Ibid., 197.

Chapter 11

26. Nikhilananda, *Vivekananda*, 614.

Chapter 14

27. Swami Kriyananda [Donald J. Walters], *Conversations with Yogananda* (Nevada City, CA: Crystal Clarity Publishers, 2004), 338.

28. Ibid., 392.

29. Ibid., 284.

Chapter 15

30. Nikhilananda, *Vivekananda*, 731–732.

Chapter 16

31. Kriyananda, *Conversations*, 119.

32. Yogananda, *God Talks*, 615.

33. Godman, *Be As You Are*, 118.

34. Yogananda, *Divine Romance*, 87.

35. Sri Chinmoy, *Meditation: Man-Perfect in God-Satisfaction* (Jamaica, NY: Aum Publications, 1989), 82.

Chapter 17

36. This reading was given in 1933. In today's currency value (2007/2008), $250,000 would equate to approximately 3.8 to 4.0 million dollars. Source: http://www.measuringworth.com/uscompare/

Chapter 18

37. Glen Sanderfur, *Lives of the Master: The Rest of the Jesus Story* (Virginia Beach, VA: A.R.E. Press, 1988), 63.

38. [The early Priestly sect that documented Enoch] strongly influenced later Hebrew notions of immortality and gave rise to a whole body of pseudigraphical literature in which Enoch is a model of divine wisdom. Stephen L. Harris and Robert L. Platzner, *The Old Testament: An Introduction to the Hebrew Bible* (New York: McGraw–Hill, 2003), G–12.

39. Harris and Platzner, *Old Testament*, 369–370.

40. Robinson, *Nag Hammadhi*, 444.

41. Harris and Platzner, *Old Testament*, 386.

42. Sanderfur, *Lives*, 126.

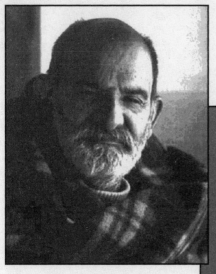

Baba Neem Karoli

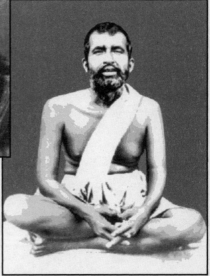

Paramahansa Ramakrishna
Photo courtesy of Ramakrishna-
Vivekananda Center of New York

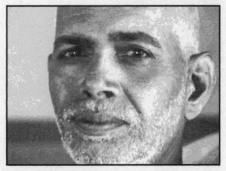

Sri Ramana Maharshi

Glossary

Word	Meaning
Adamah	Hebrew for "clay" or "earth"; commonly misunderstood as a given name in the English translation "Adam."
Ahimsa	"Non-violence" or "non-harming;" implies a commitment to actively promoting peaceful thought and behavior.
Aparigraha	Non-avarice, non-greed.
Aramaic	A northwest Semitic language that was the common vernacular at the time of Jesus; the proto-language for Hebrew and Arabic; a language found throughout the Tanakh, especially in the Books of Daniel and Ezra.
Asana	"Seat"—a posture or position of the body; the individual poses in hatha yoga.
Ashtangha	The "eightfold" path of yoga (also known in some sects as Raja Yoga): yamas, niyamas, asana, pranayama, pratyahara, dharana, dhyana, and samadhi.
Asteya	Non-stealing.

Bar Mitzvah	"Son of the commandment" – Jewish ceremony for a young man of 13 to promise to uphold the commands of the Torah.
Buddhi	"Awareness" or "wisdom"; a cognitive state above *manas*, denoting a more refined spiritual intelligence and awareness.
Christ Consciousness	The exalted spiritual consciousness that was of the historical Yeshua of ancient Palestine and many other great masters; a state of perfect self-transcendence and spiritual awareness of God; perfect egolessness in the midst of worldly service and sacrifice.
Dharana	Concentration, attention or focusing; being able to internalize and focus one's mind.
Dhyana	Meditation; the word implies effort or work.
Essene	According to the historian Josephus, one of the "four schools of thought" in ancient Judaism; according to the Cayce readings, a subset of Judaism of which both Jesus and John the Baptist's families were members; meaning "expectant," they can be traced back to the time of the biblical

Samuel as preparing themselves as channels for the Messiah.

God-realization

The authentic internal experience of enlightened mind; inner light and bliss as the natural result of disempowering the ego; a transmundane awareness of being united with the Source of the Universe.

Gnosticism

Derived from the Greek "gnosis" (knowledge), it is a collective term for various groups of esoteric religionists between the 1st and 6th centuries CE that valued mystical realization over doctrinal authority; especially proliferate in Egypt.

Isvara-pranidhana

Isvara = "God" or "Lord"—pranidhana = "under full placement" or complete surrender to; devotion to the internal Higher Self or Inner Lord.

Kriya Yoga

The yoga (union) of action; the primary exposition of the Yoga Sutras; the system of God-realization as taught by Paramahansa Yogananda and his lineage.

Mahayogi

A great yogi; one who has transcended one's ego-self to realize one's God-self.

Manas	"Mind"; the lower cognitive state, functioning primarily as a relay station for the senses; the restless and often capricious mental habits; the mind that is limited to information instead of attuned to intuitive wisdom.
Nag Hammadi	Egyptian city where in 1945 a collection of 45 Gnostic papyrus scrolls or scroll fragments were discovered.
Nirvana	"Blowing out" or "extinction"; a commonly employed term in Buddhism denoting liberation from incarnational cycles and their related states of suffering.
Niyamas	"Adherences"—the five disciplines that develop character and shape a quality citizen.
Patañjali	Author of the *Yoga Sutras* circa 200 CE; historically, there were numerous teachers writing under this name, spanning hundreds of years.
Pranayama	"Control of prana [vital energy]"— various breathing techniques meant to increase vital energy and assist in mental focus.

Pratyahara	Internal withdrawal of the senses.
Samadhi	"Putting together" or "ecstasy"—a supraconscious bliss, free from all ideational thought; an advanced state of spiritual realization.
Samskaras	Subliminal impressions derived from past–life experiences and present-life choices; these are the activating forces that often shape a personality and help explain habits and behavioral propensities.
Samyama	"Holding together"; the collective activities of dharana, dhyana, and samadhi; the highest systematic tier of Raja Yoga.
Santosha	"Contentment"—a mindset of accepting all present conditions as perfect for spiritual growth and wisdom.
Satya	"Truth"—purity of intention in thought and action.
Yamas	The moral restraints as defined by Patanjali and subsequent sages.

Bibliography

The Amplified Bible. Grand Rapids, MI: Zondervan Publishing, 1987.

Chinmoy, Sri. *Meditation: Man-Perfect in God-Satisfaction.* Jamaica, NY: Aum Publications, 1989.

Feuerstein, George. *The Yoga Tradition: Its History, Literature, Philosophy and Practice.* Prescott, AZ: Bhavana Books and Prints, 1998.

Godman, David, ed. *Be As You Are: The Teachings of Sri Ramana Maharshi.* New York: Penguin Books, 1985.

Harris, Stephen L., and Robert L. Platzner. *The Old Testament: An Introduction to the Hebrew Bible.* New York: McGraw–Hill, 2003.

Khan, Hazrat Inayat. *The Complete Sayings of Hazrat Inayat Khan.* New Lebanon, NY: Sufi Order Publications, 1978.

Kriyananda, Swami [Donald J. Walters]. *Conversations with Yogananda.* Nevada City, CA: Crystal Clarity Publishers, 2004.

Nikhilananda, Swami, comp. *Vivekananda: The Yogas and Other Works.* New York, NY: Ramakrishna–Vivekananda Center, 1984.

——, trans. *The Gospel of Sri Ramakrishna.* New York, NY: Ramakrishna–Vivekananda Center, 1984.

Prophet, Elizabeth Clare. *The Lost Years of Jesus.* Livingston, MT: Summit University Press, 1987.

Robinson, James M., ed. *The Nag Hammadhi Library,* 3rd ed. San Francisco, CA: Harper, 1988.

Sanderfur, Glen. *Lives of the Master: The Rest of the Jesus Story.* Virginia Beach,

VA: A.R.E. Press, 1988.

A Search for God, Book I. Virginia Beach, VA: A.R.E. Press, 2007.

A Search for God, Book II. Virginia Beach, VA: A.R.E. Press, 2008.

Tanakh: A New Translation of the Holy Scriptures According to the Traditional Hebrew Text. New York: The Jewish Publication Society, 1985.

Yogananda, Paramahansa. *The Divine Romance*. Los Angeles, CA: Self–Realization Fellowship, 1988.

——. *God Talks with Arjuna: The Bhagavad Gita, Royal Science of God-Realization*. Los Angeles, CA: Self–Realization Fellowship, 1995.

——. *Man's Eternal Quest*. Los Angeles, CA: Self–Realization Fellowship, 1988.

A.R.E. PRESS

EDGAR CAYCE'S A.R.E.

What Is A.R.E.?

The Association for Research and Enlightenment, Inc., (A.R.E.®) was founded in 1931 to research and make available information on psychic development, dreams, holistic health, meditation, and life after death. As an open-membership research organization, the A.R.E. continues to study and publish such information, to initiate research, and to promote conferences, distance learning, and regional events. Edgar Cayce, the most documented psychic of our time, was the moving force in the establishment of A.R.E.

Who Was Edgar Cayce?

Edgar Cayce (1877–1945) was born on a farm near Hopkinsville, Ky. He was an average individual in most respects. Yet, throughout his life, he manifested one of the most remarkable psychic talents of all time. As a young man, he found that he was able to enter into a self-induced trance state, which enabled him to place his mind in contact with an unlimited source of information. While asleep, he could answer questions or give accurate discourses on any topic. These discourses, more than 14,000 in number, were transcribed as he spoke and are called "readings."

Given the name and location of an individual anywhere in the world, he could correctly describe a person's condition and outline a regimen of treatment. The consistent accuracy of his diagnoses and the effectiveness of the treatments he prescribed made him a medical phenomenon, and he came to be called the "father of holistic medicine."

Eventually, the scope of Cayce's readings expanded to include such subjects as world religions, philosophy, psychology, parapsychology, dreams, history, the missing years of Jesus, ancient civilizations, soul growth, psychic development, prophecy, and reincarnation.

A.R.E. Membership

People from all walks of life have discovered meaningful and life-transforming insights through membership in A.R.E. To learn more about Edgar Cayce's A.R.E. and how membership in the A.R.E. can enhance your life, visit our Web site at EdgarCayce.org, or call us toll-free at 800-333-4499.

Edgar Cayce's A.R.E.
215 67th Street
Virginia Beach, VA 23451–2061

EDGARCAYCE.ORG